Clinical
Reflexology

For Elsevier
Commissioning Editor: Claire Wilson
Development Editor: Helen Leng
Project Manager: Jagannathan Varadarajan
Designer/Design Direction: Kirsteen Wright
Illustration Manager: Merlyn Harvey
Illustrator: Robert Britton

Clinical Reflexology

A guide for integrated practice

Second Edition

Edited by

Denise Tiran MSc RM RGN ADM PGCEA, reflex zone therapist
Director, Expectancy, and Visiting Lecturer,
University of Greenwich, London UK

Peter A Mackereth PhD MA RGN CertEd DipNurs
Clinical Lead for Complementary Therapy and Smoking Cessation
Services, The Christie NHS Foundation Trust, Manchester, UK

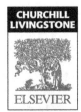

CHURCHILL
LIVINGSTONE

ELSEVIER

EDINBURGH LONDON NEW YORK OXFORD PHILADELPHIA
ST LOUIS SYDNEY TORONTO 2011

CHURCHILL LIVINGSTONE
ELSEVIER

First edition 2002
Second edition 2011

ISBN 9780702031670

British Library Cataloguing in Publication Data
A catalogue record for this book is available from the British Library

Library of Congress Cataloging in Publication Data
A catalog record for this book is available from the Library of Congress

Notices
Knowledge and best practice in this field are constantly changing. As new research and experience broaden our understanding, changes in research methods, professional practices, or medical treatment may become necessary.

Practitioners and researchers must always rely on their own experience and knowledge in evaluating and using any information, methods, compounds, or experiments described herein. In using such information or methods they should be mindful of their own safety and the safety of others, including parties for whom they have a professional responsibility.

With respect to any drug or pharmaceutical products identified, readers are advised to check the most current information provided (i) on procedures featured or (ii) by the manufacturer of each product to be administered, to verify the recommended dose or formula, the method and duration of administration, and contraindications. It is the responsibility of practitioners, relying on their own experience and knowledge of their patients, to make diagnoses, to determine dosages and the best treatment for each individual patient, and to take all appropriate safety precautions.

To the fullest extent of the law, neither the Publisher nor the authors, contributors, or editors, assume any liability for any injury and/or damage to persons or property as a matter of products liability, negligence or otherwise, or from any use or operation of any methods, products, instructions, or ideas contained in the material herein.

CONTENTS

CONTENTS

CONTRIBUTORS

Denise Tiran, MSc RM RGN ADM PGCEA, reflex zone therapist
Director, Expectancy, and Visiting Lecturer, University of Greenwich, London
Denise is an experienced midwife who practises several complementary therapies, including reflex zone therapy. She is an internationally renowned authority on maternity-related complementary medicine and has written/edited ten textbooks and over 40 journal papers; her latest book is *Reflexology for Pregnancy and Childbirth* (2010). Clinically, Denise specialises in using structural reflex zone therapy to treat women with "morning sickness" and has treated over 5000 expectant mothers in the last 25 years. Her research activities have included an investigation into using reflexology to predict stages of the female menstrual cycle. In this book, Denise explores the physiological basis of reflexology, revisits some of the "rules" of reflexology, discusses treatment for women with infertility problems and for those who are pregnant, and introduces her own modification of reflexology, termed Structural Reflex Zone Therapy.

Peter A Mackereth, PhD MA RGN CertEd DipNurs
Clinical Lead for Complementary Therapy and Smoking Cessation Services
Peter has had a varied career in nursing, teaching and research, occupying roles such as intensive care charge nurse, researcher, Senior Lecturer and university Reader. He currently works in a large cancer care unit leading a team of therapists and coordinating a programme of university accredited courses. Peter has an MA in Medical Ethics and recently completed a PhD project examining therapeutic outcomes for reflexology. In 2003 the Complementary Therapy team at the Christie received the prestigious Prince of Wales's Good Practice Award. In 2005 Peter was given the National Public Servant Award hosted by the Guardian Newspaper. Peter has published widely and speaks regularly at conferences and study days. In this book, Peter contributes his experience and understanding of the challenges of integrating this therapy, with a particular focus on the psychological basis for therapeutic outcomes of reflexology, on research and educational issues and on using reflexology for smoking cessation.

Gunnel Berry, MSc MCSP Leg.sjukgym (Sweden)
Gunnel is a chartered physiotherapist with 38 years' clinical practice, primarily in musculoskeletal outpatient domains in England, Sweden and East

Malaysia. She qualified as a reflexologist in 1989 and has developed her own methodology called "Adapted Reflextherapy", which she has presented at various international and national conferences over the last ten years. Gunnell is a member of the Health Professionals' Council; a clinical specialist in pain management; a visiting lecturer at The Christie, Manchester; external assessor for the Midland School of Reflextherapy; and Director of G Berry Ltd. In her chapter, Gunnel introduces Adapted Reflextherapy and discusses its application to the management of chronic pain, particularly in relation to whiplash injury.

Jenny Gordon, PhD RSCN
Jenny is Programme Manager, (Evidence for Practice), at the Royal College of Nursing, London. Jenny is a reflexologist and contributed aspects from her own PhD research for the chapter on teaching parents to use reflexology for their children.

Edwina Hodkinson, RGN BRCP MAR
Edwina has worked as the Clinical Lead for Complementary Therapy at Bury Cancer Centre and Deputy Clinical Lead for Complementary Therapy at The Christie Hospital. She has a background in general nursing, with qualifications in reflexology, aromatherapy and healing. Edwina has contributed to the chapter on reflexology and cancer care.

Professor Christopher Johns, RN FACT PhD
Chris is Professor of Nursing at the University of Bedfordshire, and a practising complementary therapist, Hospice of St Francis, Berkhampsted. Chris has an international reputation for his work on mindfulness in nursing and on reflective practice. His chapter introduces the reader to the use of written narrative to aid reflection in and on their personal clinical practice.

Anita Mehrez, RGN MIFPA
Anita was a sister on a Neurosciences Unit before entering into complementary therapies. She is a qualified reflexologist, hypnotherapist, aromatherapist and "No-Hands" Master practitioner. She has also provided complementary therapies to patients with advanced metastatic and non malignant diseases in their own homes. Anita is currently the deputy Clinical Lead for complementary therapy services at The Christie and has a private practice in Manchester. Anita is co-author of the reflexology and cancer care chapter.

Paula Maycock LI Biol, LI Acu MIFPA MAR
Paula is a senior therapist at the Christie NHS Foundation Trust, using an integrated approach which incorporates several therapies, including reflexology, hypnosis, aromatherapy and acupuncture. She supports her practise scientifically from her previous work in biochemistry and microbiology and from many years' experience of working with people living with long term illness. Paula is proactive in promoting and supporting the use of complementary therapies in the successful attainment of a *Smoke Free* lifestyle, and in her chapter she discusses how reflexology can be a useful adjunct to helping clients to stop smoking.

Beverly Newbury, BSc (Hons) Cert Ed MCAR, reflexologist

Beverly is a reflexology practitioner and a lecturer and programme leader for the complementary therapy degree programme at the University of Salford; she has taught practitioner training courses for over 10 years and has also been involved in the provision of continuing professional development for tutorial staff. Beverly has a small private reflexology practice and is a Council member for the Clinical Association of Reflexologists. Beverly's chapter focuses on educational issues and the need for continuing professional development.

Jill Norfolk, BSc ITEC RDHA BTER

Jill is a reflexologist and Bowen technique practitioner and teacher. She developed the Foot-applied Bowen method and now teaches this system internationally. Jill is also Director and creator of Atlantis Island Flower essences.

Helen Poole, PhD BSc (Hons)

Helen is a senior lecturer at Liverpool John Moore's University. She is a chartered psychologist and her doctoral thesis evaluated the use of reflexology for the management of chronic low back pain. Helen's chapter updates the research chapter from the first edition of *Clinical Reflexology* and examines ways in which practitioners can become involved in evaluating their own practice.

Professor Julie Stone, MA LLB Barrister

Julie is a lawyer by background and specialises in the ethical, legal and regulatory aspects of healthcare. She was appointed by the Secretary of State for Health as a lay member of the NHS Complaints Panel, and is a member of a multi-centre research ethics committee. She is a Visiting Professor of professional ethics, and lectures internationally on regulation, medico-legal issues, research ethics, and the professionalisation and regulation of complementary medicine and psychotherapy. Julie was previously the Deputy Director of the Council for Healthcare Regulatory Excellence (2003 to 2006), responsible for the implementation of regulatory change across the UK's statutory healthcare sector, and is also a non-Executive Director of a Primary Care Trust (PCT). Her chapter focuses on the legal, ethical and professional issues confronting reflexologists, especially in light of the greater integration of the therapy within conventional healthcare settings such as the NHS.

Liz Tipping, RGN RM Dip Reflex Adv Reflex

Liz worked as a nursing sister in a regional Neonatal Intensive Care Unit before taking early retirement. She practises reflexology and specialises in working with babies and children. She is an accredited infant massage teacher, has developed a neonatal massage workshop for professionals and runs courses for parents in local family centres in Wales. Liz is also a committee member (Special Needs Coordinator) for the Guild of Infant and Child Massage. In her chapter. Liz explores how reflexologists may be able to teach parents to use reflexology on their babies and children.

Julia M Williams, MIGPP MIHAF MAR

Julia practises reflexology and several other complementary therapies. She was worked in various different clinical fields and now works in cancer care. Julia contributed to the chapter on using reflexology for people living with cancer.

Jan Williamson, MAR ITEC(Hons) BWYDipCertEd
Jan is a reflexology tutor, running full professional training courses. She also teaches extensively both in the UK and abroad to qualified practitioners in the specific skills involved in Precision Reflexology. She is a yoga tutor with regular classes and specialising in pre- and post-natal and baby classes. Jan is a co-author on the chapter on incorporating new techniques.

PREFACE

We were invited to produce a new edition of *Clinical Reflexology* in response to feedback from practitioners who had been inspired by the contributions in our first edition. Since its publication the profession of reflexology has become further integrated into clinical practice, which has created more dynamic debate and interest amongst practitioners and within the wider healthcare and research communities. This second edition is a companion to the first rather than a substitute, adding to the body of knowledge available to students and practitioners of this fascinating modality.

In the pursuit of sustained integration of complementary therapies into conventional healthcare, reflexology (and other therapies) is continuing to evolve. While there is a need to identify and retain the valuable core principles of the original therapy, and ensure that these are not lost in the process, it is essential to acquire a deeper understanding of the theoretical principles. It behoves the profession of reflexology to produce critical and reflective practitioners, to acknowledge the value of remaining curious, to challenge assumptions, and to be willing to engage in research and enquiry.

In preparing this new edition of *Clinical Reflexology* we were committed to disseminate a wider critical understanding and appraisal of the therapy, to encourage others to debate objectively in order to enhance the development of the profession. In Section 1 the principle chapters have been revised and updated to emphasize the key professional issues, such as education, legal and ethical concerns and research. New elements have been included, with a focus on some of the theoretical debates related to the mechanism of action and therapeutic outcomes of reflexology, and on becoming a more reflective, accountable and inquisitive practitioner. In Section 2 we have brought together a wealth of insight, experience and expertise from a number of advanced practitioners and educators, who have contributed chapters on various clinical specialties, from preconception to end of life care.

In selecting this book we hope it will inspire you to continue to examine and develop your personal potential as a creative reflexologist; motivate, engage and sustain you in the challenge of integrating reflexology into conventional health care settings; and act as a role model for others within the profession.

Denise Tiran & Peter Mackereth 2010

ACKNOWLEDGEMENTS

The Editors would like to thank all the contributors who have worked tirelessly to bring this new work to fruition, especially in the light of all the other personal and professional challenges in their lives.

Denise would like to thank her partner, Harry Chummun, for his love and support and, particularly, for his assistance with applying physiological principles to reflexology practice in Chapter 1. As always, she would like to dedicate this book to her wonderful son, Adam, who is now 20, at university in London and soon to embark on his own career in Africa, but who still sometimes enjoys the relaxation of a reflexology treatment.

Peter would like to thank his partner, Stephen McGinn, for his unstinting support; Tom Hall for his encouragement in all things academic and, importantly, many thanks go to Dr Valerie Hillier, Dr Katie Booth and Dr Ann-Louise Caress for their support and supervision during his doctoral study.

Finally, our grateful thanks go to all the patients, students and teachers who have inspired us over the years to deepen our knowledge and skills in reflexology, and who have motivated us to share this with others.

SECTION I
PROFESSIONAL ISSUES IN CLINICAL REFLEXOLOGY

SECTION CONTENTS

INTRODUCTION

This new edition of *Clinical Reflexology* has been divided into two sections. The first consists of seven chapters, each a critical review of a contemporary theme related to clinical reflexology by authors with specific expertise on the topics examined. The areas of education, research and ethics and law are revised versions of the original chapters from the first edition. The other chapters present and develop perspectives based on evolving understandings of the theory and professional practice of reflexology. The core themes are a foundation for Section II.

All chapters begin with a short abstract and key words to aid future literature searching. There are supportive references, case studies (anonymous to protect client confidentiality) and further reading and useful resources.

Chapter 1. The physiological basis of reflexology – Denise Tiran. This chapter debates the mechanism of action of reflexology from a physiological perspective. The author emphasises the need for an understanding of physiology in relation to clinical practice of reflexology and provides a worked example to illustrate the dynamic process and outcomes.

Chapter 2. The psychological basis for therapeutic outcomes of reflexology – Peter Mackereth. This chapter explores the various psychological factors which may influence the therapeutic outcomes of reflexology. The concept of the 'healing crisis' is examined, with recommendations for informed consent and the provision of the reflexology care package.

Chapter 3. Educational developments – Beverly Newbury and Peter Mackereth. This chapter examines key developmental issues in the provision of educational courses, the importance of continuing education and the need for mentoring and supervision of ongoing practice.

Chapter 4. Ethical, legal and professional principles – Julie Stone. This chapter outlines the major ethical and legal responsibilities owed by reflexologists to their clients. The author examines the concept of duty of care and the importance of working within the law.

Chapter 5. Reflection in reflexology practice through the use of narrative – Christopher Johns. This chapter explores the potential for reflection and reflective practice to aid learning and enhance practice. It focuses on the use of narrative, which can be a useful aid to facilitate the therapist to develop sensitivity and to learn from experience.

Chapter 6. Reflexology: expanding the evidence – Helen Poole and Peter Mackereth. This chapter considers the need for research in reflexology and the questions to be asked. The authors consider research ethics, describe some common research designs with their limitations, and provide an overview of more recent studies and their findings.

Chapter 7. Revisiting the 'rules' of reflexology – Denise Tiran. This chapter explores some of the rules and traditions of reflexology and challenges their validity in contemporary clinical reflexology practice, especially when reflexology is incorporated into mainstream healthcare.

The physiological basis of reflexology

Denise Tiran

ABSTRACT

This chapter explores some of the theories on the mechanism of action of reflexology, particularly relating them to physiological actions and effects, and considering currently available research that may support these theories.

KEY WORDS

Physiology, mechanism of action, neural pathways, Schumann resonance, placebo effect, touch, meridians

INTRODUCTION

Reflexology is a therapeutic modality based on the principle that one small area of the body represents a 'map' of the whole, so that each part of the body is reflected on one or both feet, or on the hands or other area such as the tongue or ear. Reflexology has an increasingly scientific underpinning based on a deepening understanding of the physiological mechanisms of action. However, it is also an art, in which sensitivity and creativity are core and in which the basic concepts of complementary medicine – body, mind and spirit – are fundamental to the care of clients. Reflexology is a manual therapy but,

3

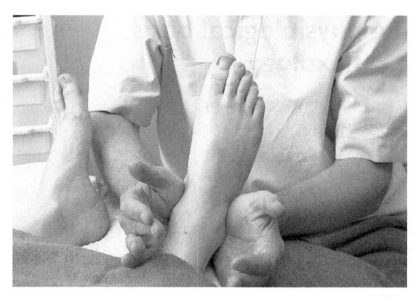

FIG. 1.1 Photo courtesy of Katie Spruce BA (Hons), medical photographer, Christie Hospital NHS Trust, with permission.

although there are similarities with other touch therapies, it is not just foot 'massage'. It has its own mechanism of action, yet to be fully clarified, identified indications, contraindications and precautions, effects, reactions and complications. There is also an emerging body of evidence, albeit relatively small compared to other therapies, but one which paves the way for further understanding and exploration of this fascinating therapy.

Reflexology originates from ancient Chinese, Indian and Egyptian techniques, and the practice reached Europe in the fourteenth century. The modern reflexology profession evolved from the early twentieth-century work of William Fitzgerald, who recognised the principle of 'zone analgesia' and investigated widely in order to define the 'maps' of the reflex points on the feet and hands. The American masseuse, Eunice Ingham, developed one of the original 'maps' and produced the first of the modern reflexology charts, while the German midwife, Hanne Marquardt, further refined the reflex zone concept. In the UK, contemporary reflexology is classified as a 'supportive' therapy (House of Lords 2000) with the implications (1) that it is a *complementary* therapy rather than one which can be used in isolation, and (2) that there is a relatively limited body of research evidence (compared to other therapies). Reflexology is progressing towards voluntary self-regulation through the Reflexology Forum, which has defined a common core curriculum and the requirements for continuing professional development of qualified practitioners (see Ch. 3).

CLAIMS FOR REFLEXOLOGY

It is claimed that reflexology helps to restore and maintain homeostasis, to be relaxing, destressing and to relieve pain, and there is much anecdotal evidence to support this. It has been said to aid circulation and excretion, reduce inflammation, balance the nervous system and even improve muscle tone, 'through nerve stimulation' (Crane 1997:xii–xv). Some consider that reflexology has the potential to assist, indirectly, in cell renewal and wound healing through increased circulation and other purported physiological effects. Reflexology treatment aims to facilitate the person's innate self-healing processes, not merely suppressing symptoms but possibly also limiting the effects of disease.

We know, from observing clients, that reflexology is a powerful relaxation tool. Clients frequently report improved sleep and experience effects of treatment such as increased excretion of urine, stools or sweat, and an improvement in the presenting condition, or a temporary resurgence of old symptoms. These reactions are considered a 'healing crisis' which allow the body to rid itself of the negative effects of disease, in order to regain homeostasis, although this theory does not appear to have been extensively researched. Reactions also occur during treatment, including temperature changes, emotional responses and tenderness in parts of the feet apparently related to the presenting condition. Experienced practitioners will also notice changes in the feet as a result of the treatments, either visually or on palpation, or the client will report symptomatic reactions to treatment.

However, what we do *not* know, at least from a scientific perspective, is precisely *how* reflexology works, its mechanism of action, how it differs from other manual therapies, and – somewhat contentiously – which reflexology 'maps' or charts are accurate. It is these aspects which need to be clarified in order to raise the credibility of the profession of reflexology, especially in the eyes of conventional healthcare practitioners. A profession is characterised by a set of specialist skills based on a specific body of knowledge, acquired through formal education and continuing professional development, with advanced practice based on research evidence where possible. However, until there is agreement amongst reflexology authorities, with standardisation of theory and practice, it will be impossible to develop reflexology further as a profession. Teachers, practitioners and academics of reflexology remain unable to agree on the precise location of many reflex points and there are numerous different charts available, a fact which has provoked considerable debate for many years (O'Hara 2002; see also Ch. 7). Whilst it is professionally acceptable – and, indeed, desirable – to have academic debate which may lead generic reflexology to evolve into many different styles, the lack of consensus about the basic principles and the theoretical background from which we all work needs to be relatively uniform. Lack of consistency between reflexology charts is akin to having different textbooks for anatomy from which student doctors can select their preferred style.

THE MECHANISM OF ACTION OF REFLEXOLOGY

Reflexology aims to treat through 'stimulation' of reflex points or zones on one small area of the body which appear to link involuntarily to others via a network of channels, neurones or transmitters. Reflexology is a touch therapy, in common with massage, shiatsu, aromatherapy or osteopathy, and many people believe that its therapeutic effects stem largely from the impact of touch in general, rather than working on any specifically identified points. Others suggest that any benefits arise from the placebo effect and/or the interaction between the client and the therapist. It is, of course, impossible to distinguish the effects of touch, nor those of the therapeutic relationship, from the overall clinical benefits of reflexology. Indeed, it is this very interaction which may make reflexology a definitive clinical modality which is distinctly different from massage or other therapies. If a client 'feels better' from having reflexology – and no harm is done – it is irrelevant, at least in human terms, how or why the treatment has led to this outcome. However, in scientific terms it is important to understand more about how reflexology works, as this will facilitate further developments and give us a deeper appreciation of indications for use, as well as contraindications and precautions for safe practice.

TOUCH

Touch, applied in a therapeutic environment in the form of massage, has been shown to aid relaxation through the release of endorphins and the neuropeptides, serotonin and dopamine, which in turn suppress the levels of the stress hormones, cortisol, epinephrine and norepinephrine (adrenaline and noradrenaline) (Field et al. 2005). High circulating levels of cortisol, in particular, lead to a reduced ability to cope with the effects of stress, an increased heart rate and blood pressure, poor sleep patterns, a greater perception of pain, more sensitivity to infections and slower wound healing from an impaired immune system and hyperglycaemia from raised blood glucose (Kirschbaum et al. 1995). Furthermore, abnormally high cortisol levels may interfere with stomach acid, causing potassium loss; this results in a rise in sodium, leading to oedema and hypertension, and to reduced muscle tone and bone density. Raised cortisol also impairs memory and the ability to learn, and seriously interferes with the functioning of numerous hormones including insulin, oestrogen, progesterone, oxytocin and thyroid hormones (Kirschbaum et al. 1996).

Massage and touch have been shown to negate some of these adverse effects, including reducing the blood pressure (BP), improving sleep patterns and enhancing immune system functioning (Field 2002), and work on preterm infants has demonstrated improved growth (Gonzalez et al. 2009), enhanced brain development and visual acuity (Guzzetta et al. 2009). Similarly, a recent study by Billhult et al. (2009) on women with breast cancer revealed a reduction in systolic BP, heart rate and natural killer (NK) cells (i.e. enhancement of the immune system). However, this study did not demonstrate any decrease in diastolic BP or cortisol levels. A systematic review of several massage studies consistently found a reduction in salivary cortisol and heart rate following single treatments, but this was not upheld significantly in those studies where multiple treatments were given (Moraska et al. 2008). Reflexology-specific trials have evaluated the effects on perceived stress, including the use of self-administered treatment for depression in middle-aged women (Lee 2006), although it is interesting to note that this study also did not reveal significant changes in cortisol or diastolic BP from repeated self-administration. Another investigation of 'reflexology foot massage' by Song and Kim (2006) demonstrated a significant improvement in sleep patterns in the elderly, together with an (expected) increase in serotonin levels. Similar results were demonstrated with reflexology for postpartum women (Li et al. 2009) but, in both these studies, successful outcomes may have been achieved from the impact of touch in general, rather than reflexology in particular.

The analgesic effect of manual pressure has also been well researched, and is thought to be due partly to activation of opioid pathways which decrease nociceptive transmission of pain (the 'gate control' theory) (Jain et al. 2006). Pain relief may result from an increase in endorphins in the blood and possibly also in the brain and cerebrospinal fluid, or analgesia may simply be due to raised temperature in the peripheral tissues (Bender et al. 2007). Several controlled studies have shown that massage can relieve headache (Moraska & Chandler 2008) and acute post-operative pain (Mitchinson et al. 2007), alleviate discomfort and muscle fatigue after excessive exercise (Frey Law et al. 2008; Ogai et al. 2008) and offer short-term relief for chronic pain (Seers et al. 2008). To investigate the physiological pathways by which this analgesia occurs, Sager et al. (2007) used magnetic resonance imaging to study the effects of soft tissue changes, and found that massage has a direct effect on local fascia, muscles and nerves, and a delayed effect on the subcortical central nervous system. One specific study on the analgesic effects of reflexology showed a reduction in the duration and intensity of phantom limb pain in amputees (Brown & Lido 2008), although again, the impact of touch and the client–therapist interaction cannot be ruled out. A case study report of two cancer patients highlighted successful analgesia with a combination of reflexology and music (Magill & Berenson 2008), but in this study relief of pain cannot be assumed to be due solely to the reflexology.

It is also impossible to dismiss the impact of the placebo effect and the therapeutic relationship between the client and the reflexologist. However, since neither touch nor placebo is an exclusive facet of reflexology, this factor does not explain the apparent success of reflexology in treating specific conditions. In addition, reflexology frequently elicits in clients various signs and symptoms which appear to be responses to treatment, including some responses which do not normally occur with massage alone. There is, however, relatively limited research on reflexology, much of which incurs some criticism of the methodology, the majority of studies being neither randomised nor controlled, nor accounting for the effects of placebo or interaction between the therapist and client.

The specific mechanism of action of reflexology has traditionally been attributed by practitioners to the effects of 'stimulation' of the numerous nerve endings in the feet with manual pressure, thought to link with other areas of the body, particularly in relation to stress, since stress patterns are thought to manifest on the feet. The intensity of pressure applied during a reflexology treatment may be significant, depending on which types of sensory nerve receptors in the skin are stimulated, although positive effects have been achieved using styles of reflexology in which different pressures are employed, e.g. reflex zone therapy versus precision or Morrell reflexology. When the skin is touched, the cells emit an electrical current (an 'action potential'), and sensory nerves transmit this to the brain, from where it is relayed to local muscles for a response. Touch, pressure, temperature and stimulation of different types of receptors influence the speed of nerve transmission and the overall stimulatory effect, which can be measured via special technical apparatus, possibly, in the future, enabling us to identify the precise physiological pathways by which these impulses become effective (Makina & Shinoda 2004; Ascari et al. 2007).

NEURAL PATHWAY RELATIONSHIP

Proponents of reflex zone therapy suggest that the mechanism of action may be related to reflex signs, referred pain and trigger points. Referred pain is a concept first described in the late nineteenth century, by the neurologist Sir Henry Head, who recognised the reflex signs of disease, in which manifestations of internal dysfunction can be observed externally. Internal organs do not have a comprehensive pain receptor system; therefore, because impaired organs cannot transmit pain impulses to conscious areas of the brain, they transmit messages to areas of skin supplied by spinal nerves (dermatomes), subcutaneous tissues and muscles in the related spinal segments. This causes either increased or decreased sensitivity to pain conveyed by nerve impulses between the skin and the organs. Autonomic nervous system changes occur as a result of disease, sometimes producing pain at a point distal to the affected organ, for example shoulder pain in the case of gall bladder disease. Stimulation of the skin causes unconscious transmission of afferent nerve impulses to internal organs, and reflex signs, mediated via the autonomic nervous system, occur in the presence of disease.

Trigger points occur in skeletal muscle, are associated with palpable hyper-irritable nodules in muscle fibres, and become sensitive to pressure via kinetic chains (Lavelle et al. 2007). An active trigger point causes referred pain elsewhere in the body through transmission of impulses along nerve pathways; a latent trigger point may result in reduced muscle coordination and balance through muscle activation patterns. Muscular pain and spasm result from a local or distant stimulus, thereby activating a myofascial trigger point in the spine, and the subsequent formation of painful secondary trigger points, which, in turn, radiate to more distal trigger points. When disease develops, activation of peripheral nerve receptors in the skin and muscle sends pain impulses to the brain (Kellgren 1938; 1939 cited in Baldry 2005). Pain can be eliminated or reduced through stimulation of cutaneous and subcutaneous receptors by activating encephalinergic inhibitory interneurons in the dorsal horn (Soloman 2002; Luo & Wang 2008), similar to the 'gate control' theory of pain relief (Melzack & Wall 1965).

SCHUMANN RESONANCE

Schumann resonance refers to the frequency of the earth's vibration, resulting from the tension existing between the earth, which has a negative electrical energy, and the positively charged ionosphere. These weak electromagnetic fields are believed to interact with the body's own electrical brainwave system (Rubik 2002). Altered alpha brainwave activity arising from ill health may cause dissonance in the balance of electrical wave transmission from the ground to the brain in an attempt to equalise the wavelength, possibly causing congestion in the feet and thereby affecting their ability to transmit energy from the ground (Laurence et al. 2000; Osman 2000). In common with acupuncture, reflexology is believed to improve the body's electromagnetic energy balance (Popp 2008) via a 'sympathetic resonance' of energy exchange between the recipient and the therapist. Measurable energy is conducted from the therapist, who is deemed to be healthy, with normal energy levels, to the client whose compromised health results in lower energy levels, until a homeostatic balance is achieved (Zhang 1995). On the other hand, if a practitioner feels tired or unwell the energy is reversed, potentially leaving the client feeling unrefreshed, whereas the practitioner may feel energised, having taken on board some of the more positive energy from the client.

MERIDIAN THEORY

Until recently, there has been no proof supporting the notion that specific points on the feet link directly to the named body part, according to the usual 'maps' or charts and Ernst's 2009 systematic review maintains that there is still no convincing evidence for its effect on any specific condition. However, a study by Nakamura et al. (2008) in which functional magnetic resonance imaging was used to detect somatosensory effects appeared to indicate a link between cortical activity and stimulation of reflex points on the feet corresponding to the shoulders, eyes and small intestines. This is an exciting study given that it is specific to reflexology whereas, hitherto, reflexologists have been constrained to applying the findings from acupuncture studies demonstrating links between one part of the body and another. Some styles of reflexology focus on the meridian approach; others use a more anatomical approach to mapping of the feet, as in reflex zone therapy (see Ch. 7; Tiran 2009).

Thus, while acupuncture research can contribute to our overall understanding, it does not adequately reflect the mechanism of action of reflexology in general, and there are some fundamental differences between reflexology and acupuncture. A practitioner of acupuncture or acupressure will work on numerous meridians and tsubos (acupuncture focus points) around the whole body, whereas reflexologists usually concentrate on the feet, hands and/or ears. Reflexologists who use the meridian approach apply treatment via the end points of those meridians which originate or terminate in the feet or hands, rather than via the conventional reflex zones and points. On the other hand, auricular acupuncture could be said to be similar to reflexology in that it uses one small area of the body (the ears) as a microcosm of the whole.

However, a link with the meridians of acupuncture is worthy of exploration. Many acupuncture points are tender to touch and may become more so in the presence of ill health, although a study by Janovsky et al. (2000) appeared to refute this. In reflexology, systemic healing is achieved by treating the relevant reflex point(s) with distal stimulation transmitted via the extracellular matrix around the body. The relationship between trigger points (see above) and acupuncture points is increasingly being investigated (Birch 2003; Kao et al. 2006), together with the neurological stimulation which occurs when acupuncture needles are inserted at points distal to the affected area (Dung et al. 2004). Langevin and Yandow (2002) demonstrated an 80% correlation between acupuncture points and interstitial connective tissue. Further, acupuncture points are known to have lower electrical resistance than the skin adjacent to them, although a systematic review of several trials challenged the methodology of this study and suggested a need for further investigations (Ahn et al. 2008). Silberstein (2009) takes this theory one step further by suggesting that acupuncture points occur where C fibre afferent nerve axons bifurcate, the fibres then diverging to run along the meridians. These subsequently communicate with Merkel cells in the skin, which have synaptic contacts with somatosensory afferent nerves and are associated with the discrimination of the shapes and textures of light touch. Commonly, Merkel cells occur in the basal skin layer at the bottom of sweat duct ridges and – interestingly – are found particularly in the invaginated skin ridges on the plantar surfaces of the feet. It is thought that inserting needles or applying pressure at the acupuncture points disrupts the bifurcation of the axons, preventing neural transmission between Merkel cells and central communication with the spinal cord.

SAFE PRACTICE

From this discussion, it is fair to acknowledge that we do not, as yet, fully understand the mechanism of action of reflexology and there remains uncertainty about which, if any, of the contemporary theories is accurate. It may be that reflexology works through a combination approach, in which the link between reflex points and other parts of the body is partly anatomical, partly energetic and partly due to extraneous factors. It is recognised by practitioners that the effects of reflexology go beyond mere touch, and there are numerous accounts in the literature of its apparent effectiveness in relieving specific symptoms or conditions. However, since many conditions explored in the research to date have an emotional component (stress, anxiety, etc.), the psychological impact of treatment cannot be disregarded and may, indeed, play a fundamental role in the mechanism of action (see Ch. 2).

Safe practice depends on a thorough understanding of reflexology, which is up to date and, where possible, based on available research evidence. Empirical data provide a reasonable body of information to support our work and enable us to collate any reports of apparent adverse effects or complications arising from inappropriate treatment, given inadvertently through lack of knowledge and an ability to apply theory to practice. Precautions and contraindications can be identified, based on knowledge derived from investigation and observation, and professional practice requires practitioners to adhere to these clinical guidelines in order to protect both their clients and themselves. It is preferable – and ethical – to work ultracautiously with some clients rather than to take a maverick and potentially dangerous approach in the misguided belief that this 'natural' therapy is completely safe. It is impossible to state, on the one hand, that reflexology aids certain physiological processes and may contribute to relief of symptoms in specific conditions, yet on the other to claim that it will not cause adverse or inappropriate effects. Either reflexology does *something* or it does *nothing* – and if it does *something* we need to know when a particular therapeutic action would be unsafe. Used professionally, reflexology should not cause undesirable complications (different from reactions to treatment) – but overzealous or poorly trained practitioners may risk performing a 'treatment' which is inappropriate, inaccurate and dangerous.

It is necessary to have a good knowledge of physiology and anatomy when performing reflexology for clinical purposes; those who do not possess a sophisticated level of knowledge have no place in clinical reflexology and are merely performing 'salon reflexology', probably giving much the same treatment to each client. Further, when treating clients with specific conditions, it is essential to understand the pathology related to their conditions, and to apply this knowledge to the individual so that treatment can be effective and safe. In addition, the practitioner must possess an adequate understanding of the potential interaction of reflexology with any conventional treatment, be it pharmacological, surgical or radiological.

In order to appreciate this interlinking of theory and practice, let us look at a worked example, in this case exploring the condition of backache in pregnancy (see also Ch. 9 and Tiran 2009). This condition has been chosen deliberately since many readers may not have wide experience of treating pregnant women, but similar worked examples could be given for other clinical specialities, featuring clients with conditions such as breast cancer or Parkinson's disease.

A WORKED EXAMPLE: LOW BACKACHE IN PREGNANCY

During pregnancy, raised cortisol levels occurring due to stress, anxiety, fear and pain can cause a variety of physiological and pathological effects. Cortisol is produced by the adrenal glands and is controlled by the pituitary gland, which also releases oxytocin. Oxytocin is an extremely significant hormone in that it is responsible for aspects of sexual response, the menstrual cycle, fertility, pregnancy, labour and the postnatal period. It increases sperm production in men and assists ovulation in women; during orgasm, oxytocin causes contraction of the vaginal and cervical muscles to suck the sperm into the uterus in an attempt to facilitate conception. During pregnancy, oxytocin aids placental circulation, and during labour it stimulates contractions, relaxes the perineum in readiness for the expulsion of the fetus and contributes to relief of pain. Immediately after the birth of the baby, it controls maternal bleeding and later aids in the establishment of lactation.

One early effect of raised cortisol levels is excessive insomnia and consequent tiredness, which in turn reduces the woman's coping abilities to respond to the normal physiological symptoms of pregnancy, including 'morning sickness' and backache. Excessive vomiting can impair thyroid function, exacerbating tiredness, thus setting up a vicious circle from which it is difficult to escape. The initial stress effects continue and may lead to hypertension and the possibility of pre-eclampsia. The impact of raised cortisol on the immune system, which is already compromised by the upheaval of pregnancy, results in an increased tendency to infections such as in the urinary tract which, if severe or not treated promptly, can lead to preterm labour. Conversely, since cortisol suppresses oxytocin, the labour hormones fail to increase sufficiently to trigger the onset of labour contractions, leading to prolonged pregnancy, with the possibility of medical induction of labour, which in itself can initiate iatrogenic complications. High circulating cortisol adversely affects muscle tone, resulting in the fetus potentially assuming a position which is not conducive to normal birth, for example breech presentation (bottom first). It also causes potassium depletion leading to oedema, and interferes with glucose metabolism, which can predispose the mother to gestational diabetes mellitus and further complications during pregnancy and birth, and for the newborn baby.

We have seen that touch and reflexology can reduce cortisol (Acolet et al. 1993; Field et al. 2005) and it has been shown to have a positive effect on onset, progress and outcome of pregnancy and birth. At the very least, one may assume that reflexology could be a valuable aid to relief of backache in pregnancy, but treatment must be based on an evaluation of the individual mother and a conclusion that it is safe to treat her. However, whilst low (sacral) backache is an extremely common physiological consequence of the relaxation effect on the pelvic joints of circulating progesterone, a differential diagnosis must be made to exclude other, pathological, causes of the backache. Depending on the precise location and nature of the mother's pain, backache may also be due to urinary tract infection, associated with constipation or be a symptom of early (premature) labour if it occurs before 37 weeks of pregnancy.

Having ascertained that the backache is physiological and warrants reflexology treatment, a decision must be made about the exact techniques to be used. Many reflexologists would give a general relaxation treatment, which in itself can be relaxing and indirectly ease discomfort and promote coping abilities. However, in clinical reflexology, notably reflex zone therapy, it is normal to take this to the next level by giving a treatment aimed at dealing with the specific presenting problem (although complete resolution will not occur until after delivery). Sedating techniques are normal for relieving pain and this can be performed on the reflex zones of the spine which are relevant to the mother's condition, whereas stimulating techniques or massage used over the reflex zones for the spine may exacerbate the problem. However, it should not be assumed that the only zones to be treated are those corresponding to the location of the pain, because this may not be the origin of the problem. For example, although most mothers experience pain in the lumbar and sacral regions of the spine, the cause may originate from a thoracic or cervical vertebra, especially if there has been any previous history of back problems. Similarly, the interconnection between the spine and other parts of the musculoskeletal system should lead the practitioner to consider the appropriateness of treating reflex zones for other areas such as the hips, sacroiliac joints, symphysis pubis or shoulders.

CONCLUSION

In the above worked example, we can see that an understanding of pregnancy physiology, an awareness of potential pathology and knowledge of the research on the effects of reflexology can be applied to the treatment of a pregnant client with backache, offering safe, appropriate and evidence-based therapy. If the practitioner wished to consider treatment of a woman with nausea associated with medical interventions for breast cancer, it would be necessary to be cognisant of the pathology of tumours developing in the breast, possible complications and routes by which the disease could spread and conventional medical treatments and their effects. This knowledge would then need to be applied to the reflexology treatment of the client, taking into account our contemporary understanding of reflexology and its mechanism of action. Similar exercises could be undertaken for treating other clients, both those seeking treatment for general health and well-being, and those with more specific pathological conditions.

It is no longer acceptable for reflexologists to offer standard treatments with little variations between clients, using the excuse that it is a natural therapy and therefore safe. If we are to believe – and increasingly to have evidence – that reflexology is a powerful tool, we need to understand it better in order to practice safely and appropriately. Working towards a greater appreciation of the mechanism of action and its physiological effects is paramount, so that we can progress reflexology as a profession and for that profession to take its rightful place in the healthcare arena.

Acolet, D., Modi, N., Giannakoulopoulos, X., Bond, C., Weg, W., Clow, A., et al., 1993. Changes in plasma cortisol and catecholamine concentrations in response to massage in preterm infants. Arch. Dis. Child. 68 (1 Spec No), 29–31.

Ahn, A.C., Colbert, A.P., Anderson, B.J., Martinsen, O.G., Hammerschlag, R., Cina, S., et al., 2008. Electrical properties of acupuncture points and meridians: a systematic review. Bioelectromagnetics 29 (4), 245–256.

Ascari, L., Corradi, P., Beccai, L., Laschi, C., 2007. A miniaturized and flexible optoelectronic sensing system for tactile skin. J Micromech. Microeng. 17, 2288–2298.

Baldry, P.E., 2005. Acupuncture, trigger points and musculoskeletal pain, third ed. Elsevier, Edinburgh, Ch 4, pp. 31–36.

Bender, T., Nagy, G., Barna, I., Tefner, I., Kádas, E., Géher, P., 2007. The effect of physical therapy on beta-endorphin levels. Eur. J. Appl. Physiol. 100 (4), 371–382.

Billhult, A., Lindholm, C., Gunnarsson, R., Stener-Victorin, E., 2009. The effect of massage on immune function and stress in women with breast cancer – a randomized controlled trial. Auton. Neurosci. Apr 17.

Birch, S., 2003. Trigger point – acupuncture point correlations revisited. J. Altern. Complement. Med. 9 (1), 91–103.

Brown, C.A., Lido, C., 2008. Reflexology treatment for patients with lower limb amputations and phantom limb pain – an exploratory pilot study. Complement. Ther. Clin. Pract. 14 (2), 124–131.

Crane, B., 1997. Reflexology: the definitive practitioner's manual. Element, London.

Dung, H., Vlogston, C.P., Dunn, J.W., 2004. Acupuncture – an anatomical approach. CRC Press, London.

Ernst, E., 2009. Is reflexology an effective intervention? A systematic review of randomised controlled trials. Med. J. Aust. 191 (5), 263–266.

Field, T., 2002. Massage therapy. Med. Clin. North Am. 86 (1), 163–171.

Field, T., Hernandez-Reif, M., Diego, M., Schanberg, S., Kuhn, C., 2005. Cortisol decreases and serotonin and dopamine increase following massage therapy. Int. J. Neurosci. 115 (10), 1397–1413.

Frey Law, L.A., Evans, S., Knudtson, J., Nus, S., Scholl, K., Sluka, K.A., 2008. Massage reduces pain perception and hyperalgesia in experimental muscle pain: a randomized, controlled trial. J. Pain, May.

Gonzalez, A.P., Vasquez-Mendoza, G., García-Vela, A., Guzmán-Ramirez, A., Salazar-Torres, M., Romero-Gutierrez, G., 2009. Weight gain in preterm infants following parent-administered Vimala massage: a randomized controlled trial. Am. J. Perinatol. 26 (4), 247–252.

Guzzetta, A., Baldini, S., Bancale, A., Baroncelli, L., Ciucci, F., Ghirri, P., et al., 2009. Massage accelerates brain development and the maturation of visual function. J. Neurosci. 29 (18), 6042–6051.

House of Lords Select Committee on Science and Technology, 2000. Sixth report on complementary and alternative medicine. HMSO, London.

Jain, S., Kumar, P., McMillan, D.D., 2006. Prior leg massage decreases pain responses to heel stick in preterm babies. J. Paediatr. Child Health 42 (9), 505–508.

Janovsky, B., White, A.R., Filshie, J., Hart, A., Ernst, E., 2000. Are acupuncture points tender? A blinded study of spleen 6. J. Altern. Complement. Med. 6 (2), 149–155.

Kao, M.J., Hsieh, Y.L., Kuo, F.J., Hong, C.Z., 2006. Electrophysiological assessment of acupuncture points. Am. J. Phys. Med. Rehabil. 85 (5), 443–448.

Kellgren, J.H., 1938. Observations on referred pain arising from muscle. Clin. Sci. 3, 175–190. In: Baldry, P.E. (Ed.), 2005. Acupuncture, trigger points and musculoskeletal pain, third ed. Elsevier, Edinburgh, Ch 4, pp. 31–36.

Kellgren, J.H., 1939. On the distribution of pain arising from deep somatic structures with charts of segmental pain areas. Clin. Sci. 4, 35–46. In: Baldry, P.E. (Ed.), 2005. Acupuncture, trigger points and musculoskeletal pain, third ed. Elsevier, Edinburgh, Ch 4, pp. 31–36.

Kirschbaum, C., Prussner, J.C., Stone, A.A., Federenko, I., Gaab, J., Lintz, D., et al., 1995. Persistent high cortisol responses to repeated psychological stress in a subpopulation of healthy men. Psychosom. Med. 57 (5), 468–474.

Kirschbaum, C., Wolf, O.T., May, M., Wippich, W., Hellhammer, D.H., 1996.

13

Stress- and treatment-induced elevations of cortisol levels associated with impaired declarative memory in healthy adults. Life Sci. 58 (17), 1475–1483.

Langevin, H.M., Yandow, J.A., 2002. Relationship of acupuncture points and meridians to connective tissue planes. Anat. Rec. 269 (6), 257–265.

Laurence, J.A., French, P.W., Lindner, R.A., McKenzie, D.R., 2000. Biological effects of electromagnetic fields – mechanisms for the effects of pulsed microwave radiation on protein conformation. J. Theor. Biol. 206 (2), 291–298.

Lavelle, E.D., Lavelle, W., Smith, H.S., 2007. Myofascial trigger points. Anesthesiol. Clin. 25 (4), 841–851.

Lee, Y.M., 2006. Effect of self-foot reflexology massage on depression, stress responses and immune functions of middle aged women. Taehan Kanho Hakhoe Chi 36 (1), 179–188.

Li, C.Y., Chen, S.C., Li, C.Y., Gau, M.L., Huang, C.M., 2009. Randomised controlled trial of the effectiveness of using foot reflexology to improve quality of sleep amongst Taiwanese postpartum women. Midwifery Jul 3.

Luo, F., Wang, J.Y., 2008. Modulation of central nociceptive coding by acupoint stimulation. Neurochem. Res. 33 (10), 1950–1955.

Makino, Y., Shinoda, H., 2004. Selective stimulation to skin receptors by suction pressure control. SICE Annual Conference Proceedings 3, 2103–2108.

Magill, L., Berenson, S., 2008. The conjoint use of music therapy and reflexology with hospitalized advanced-stage cancer patients and their families. Palliat. Support. Care 6 (3), 289–296.

Melzack, R., Wall, P.D., 1965. Pain mechanisms: A new theory. Science 150, 971–979.

Mitchinson, A.R., Kim, H.M., Rosenberg, J.M., Geisser, M., Kirsh, M., Cikrit, D., et al., 2007. Acute postoperative pain management using massage as an adjuvant therapy: a randomized trial. Arch. Surg. 142 (12), 1158–1167.

Moraska, A., Chandler, C., 2008. Changes in clinical parameters in patients with tension-type headache following massage therapy: A pilot study. J. Man. Manip. Ther. 16 (2), 106–112.

Moraska, A., Pollini, R.A., Boulanger, K., Brooks, M.Z., Teitlebaum, L., 2008. Physiological adjustments to stress measures following massage therapy: a review of the literature. Evid. Based Complement. Alternat. Med. May 7.

Nakamaru, T., Miura, N., Fukushima, A., Kawashima, R., 2008. Somatotopical relationships between cortical activity and reflex areas in reflexology: a functional magnetic resonance imaging study. Neurosci. Lett. 448 (1), 6–9.

Ogai, R., Yamane, M., Matsumoto, T., et al., 2008. Effects of petrissage massage on fatigue and exercise performance following intensive cycle pedalling. Br. J. Sports Med. Apr 2.

O'Hara, C., 2002. Challenging the 'rules' of reflexology. In: Mackereth, P., Tiran, D. (Eds.), Clinical reflexology: a guide for health professionals. Elsevier, Edinburgh, Chapter 3, pp. 33–52.

Osman, J.L., 2000. Energy medicine: the scientific basis. Churchill Livingstone, Edinburgh.

Popp, F.A., 2008. Principles of complementary medicine in terms of a suggested scientific basis. Indian J. Exp. Biol. 46 (5), 378–383.

Rubik, B., 2002. The biofield hypothesis: its biophysical basis and role. Med. J. Alternat. Complement. Med. 8 (6), 703–717.

Sagar, S.M., Dryden, T., Myers, C., 2007. Research on therapeutic massage for cancer patients: potential biologic mechanisms. J. Soc. Integr. Oncol. Fall 5 (4), 155–162.

Seers, K., Crichton, N., Martin, J., Coulson, K., Carroll, D., 2008. A randomised controlled trial to assess the effectiveness of a single session of nurse-administered massage for short-term relief of chronic non-malignant pain. BMC Nurs. 7, 10.

Silberstein, M., 2009. The cutaneous intrinsic visceral afferent nervous system: a new model for acupuncture analgesia. J. Theor. Biol. Sep 15.

Solomon, S., 2002. A review of mechanisms of response to pain therapy: why voodoo works. Headache 42 (7), 656–662.

Song, R.H., Kim, D.H., 2006. The effects of foot reflexion massage on sleep disturbance, depression disorder, and the physiological index of the elderly. Taehan Kanho Hakhoe Chi 36 (1), 15–24.

Tiran, D., 2009. Reflexology for pregnancy and childbirth; a definitive guide for healthcare professionals. Elsevier, Edinburgh.

Zhang, C.L., 1995. Acupuncture system and electromagnetic standing wave inside the body. Nature 17 (4), 52–62.

The psychological basis for therapeutic outcomes of reflexology

2

Peter Mackereth

ABSTRACT

In this chapter the various psychological factors which may influence the therapeutic outcomes of reflexology are explored. The concept of the 'healing crisis' is examined, and recommendations are made regarding 'informed consent' and the provision of the reflexology care package. Importantly, it is argued that, because reflexology creates a space and an interactive process for disclosure of worries and concerns, practitioners should be mindful of their professional boundaries, the need to develop and refine interpersonal skills, and sources of appropriate support.

KEY WORDS

Expectations, therapeutic, relationship, placebo, nocebo, reflexology-related disclosures, reflexology package.

INTRODUCTION

It may appear artificial and, indeed, contrary to a philosophy of holism, to examine the physiological and psychology bases for reflexology in two sepa-rate chapters (see Ch. 1). However, it is hoped that deconstructing the theories in this manner will encourage further debate and exploration of the practice of reflexology. In a Department of Health document, aimed at informing primary

DOI: 10.1016/B978-0-7020-3167-0.00002-0

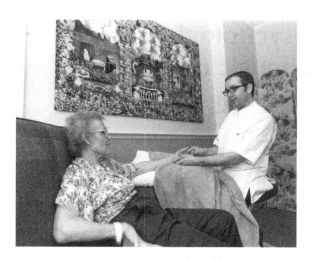

FIG. 2.1 Patient receiving hand reflexology in a relaxation room. *Reproduced with permission from Mackereth P. Journal of Complementary Therapies in Nursing and Midwifery 1999; 5(3):68.*

care groups about complementary therapies, reflexology was described as the application of pressure to the feet and/or hands in order to 'promote well-being' (DoH et al. 2000:37) (Fig. 2.1). We know that 'well-being' is so much more than just physical health, and it will be seen from the reflexology literature that well-being outcomes can be both emotional and physical (see Ch. 6). It could be argued that physical changes may primarily be a consequence of psychological processes and, given the complexity of reflexology practice, it is suggested that these are likely to be working in synergy.

Moderate amounts of stress and anxiety are a normal part of everyday life and a stimulus for activity and change. Temporary challenges to feeling good, just 'fine' and even normal can arise from marked anxiety and distress, as well as other strong emotional states, such as anger, disgust, panic and fear, which activate the sympathetic nervous division of the autonomic nervous system (ANS). Over time, persistent and unresolved anxiety and distress can cause an increase in muscle tension (tonus), reduction in peripheral skin temperatures and a hyperactive response to further recurrence of an acute stressor. The individual can have difficulty in being able to return to, or maintaining, a relaxed or calm state. The physical manifestations of chronic states of arousal and low thresholds to stressors can be seen in measurements of sympathetic nervous system (SNS) responses and physical complaints, including hypertension, impaired circulation, back and neck stiffness, digestive, bowel and skin problems. At the centre of the arguments in this chapter are the links between mind and body, which we will explore using psychoneuroimmunology (PNI) and other psychological theories.

In crossing the territory between body and mind, physiological consequences have been identified as a response to stressful situations. For example, fear can trigger changes in blood pressure and heart rate in preparation for 'flight or fight'. Arousal of the sympathetic division of the ANS can become a frequently experienced state, making the individual vulnerable to serious illness, such as myocardial infarction and peptic ulceration. It has been shown that it is possible to influence the ANS through such practices as yoga and meditation, by allowing the parasympathetic division to reduce the heart rate and blood pressure and to normalise digestive processes (Sutherland & Cooper 1995). The links between the emotional state, disease processes and experience have been – and continue to be – investigated within the scientific field of psychoneuroimmunology (PNI) (Ader 1975, 1982). The theoretical basis of PNI is that there is a two-way relationship between the immune system and the central nervous system (Rabin et al. 1989; Lloyd 1990). In understanding PNI, Carter (1998) argues that feelings of social isolation and anxiety are associated with increased stress hormones, such as cortisol.

Where moderate states of arousal and opportunities for positive social interaction and attachment coexist, physiological anxiolytic states can be created. Anxiety is central to a map of other symptoms/conditions, including insomnia, pain, depression, constipation, skin problems, irritable bowel syndrome, muscle tension, etc. If anxiety can be reduced, this will influence our tolerance and even our experience of a symptom. Improved mood and humour and relief of anxiety are linked with the release of the naturally occurring opiates, endorphins, which are believed to optimise immune function and to have analgesic, anti-inflammatory bronchodilatory effects (Jessop 2002). Opioid production is higher in individuals who exercise regularly and low in individuals who live with chronic fatigue syndrome (Conti et al. 1998). Stress hormones such as cortisol play an important part in protecting the body and sustaining fight or flight – for example, diverting blood from the gut to powerful muscles, raising blood sugar levels for energy and initiating a protective immunological response. It is when these hormones are chronically elevated that they have deleterious effects on resistance to disease and infection.

REFLEXOLOGY: THE PACKAGE AND THE MAP

There are several schools of thought regarding the mechanism of action of reflexology including an Eastern theory, whereby treatment areas relate to acupuncture meridians and 'chi' energy flow, and a Western theory, that helping to relax and destress the recipient supports their innate ability to self-heal (see Ch. 1). In deconstructing the psychological processes, it is important to recognise that reflexology, in common with other touch-based complementary and alternative medical interventions, is carried out within a one-to-one encounter, usually requiring regular appointments which aid the establishment and growth of a supportive and social relationship. Sessions typically involve hands-on treatment lasting between 35 and 50 minutes, and may include cleaning the feet and applying a small amount of moisturising cream or oil, if the feet are dry. This physical contact and the holding and relaxing manoeuvres used by the therapist mean that she or he is literally holding *the person* through the feet (Fig. 2.2). O'Hara (2002) argued that this combination of activities presents reflexology as a complex package rather than as a simple mechanical technique. Reflexology is also a journey or process, which encompasses privacy and a sense of intimacy in the interactions; time is spent with another person to help promote relaxation and improve wellbeing. The semi-recumbent position of the client facilitates face-to-face contact and conversation, which includes feedback on the pressure used as well

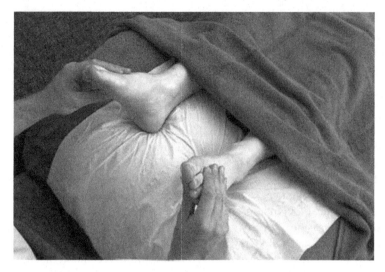

FIG. 2.2 Holding the feet – holding the person.

as opportunities for dialogue regarding the client's condition and treatment expectations. With repeated treatments, there is clearly the potential for reflexology to evolve as a supportive and social event. The intervention requires the client to put aside time, to allow himself or herself to be touched and to expect health benefits. However, with any regular contact, particularly if it is perceived as beneficial and nurturing, attachment can occur over time and it is important to recognise emerging relationships and to prevent them from becoming muddled with other types of 'being with' someone, such as becoming a friend or seeking to parent or wanting a parent to look after us. These complexities will be revisited later in the chapter.

Integral to the 'reflexology package' and which differentiates the treatment from a foot massage is a map or chart of the feet, which reflexologists use to guide their treatment. Interestingly, authors of various reflexology texts often differ on precise locations of reflex zones on the various maps (O'Hara 2002; Tiran 2009). The anatomical and physiological processes of the body can be a mystery for many people, who may have a resistance to talking about what occurs beneath the skin. Reflexologists claim that there are reflex areas on the feet, hands and ears, believed to be microcosms of the body. Both feet are palpated using thumb and finger pressure, pressing on all areas of the feet and focusing on specific areas of the feet that are tender or sensitive, which creates opportunities for interaction between a 'reflexology expert' and the person – and engagement in a journey with someone who is perceived, rightly or wrongly, to have specialist knowledge, skills and experience. The reflexology expert is also being curious about the client, who has more than likely come with concerns, and is seeking (and often paying for) skilled support, help and answers to his or her problems. The session ends with some ritualistic techniques such as 'solar plexus' breathing. Patients are usually advised to attend a minimum of six sessions, as benefits are argued to be cumulative and the repeated interactions enable further investigation, nurturing and support which all focus on the individual.

The practitioner's demeanour, willingness to listen, and use of 'quality time' may be conducive to developing a potent therapeutic relationship, and to influencing client responses (Wall & Wheeler 1996). Emotional reactions to a series of treatments are not uncommon in bodywork, and the nurturing use of touch and the support and acceptance that evolve in the therapeutic relationship may tacitly give permission for this. Additionally, these various aspects of the package can contribute to patients sharing worries and concerns, particularly about their health (Dryden et al. 1999; Mackereth 1999). Investigative work on the potential of the reflexology package for eliciting worries and concerns and affecting psychological and physical outcomes is central to the position taken in this chapter (Mackereth et al. 2009a, b).

Reflexology can be classified as a bodywork intervention with the majority of time spent in the session dedicated to the therapeutic use of touch. Montagu (1971) has argued that touch is essential for the healthy development of the individual, and provides, even in adulthood, reassurance and affirmation that an individual is accepted, valued and needed by others. Touch is a complex intervention, which can arouse numerous responses in the individual. The tactile nature of the skin is not only a means of connecting but also of differentiating between the 'me' which is inside the body and that 'which is not me' which is outside the body. The phrase 'skin ego' has its origins in Freud's comment about the body ego being a mental projection of the body's surface (Freud 1923). Reich, a student of Freud and a pioneer of body psychotherapy, identified in the 1940s that a mother's physical presence, smell and skin can moderate a child's anxiety and distress. It has been suggested that being physically present and working through touch can enable a client, even when an adult, 'to receive oneself' to gain insight, possibly to become emotional and expressive, and then to experience a sense of calmness after working through these processes (Carroll 2002). Cameron (2002) describes this experience as 'proprioception', which enables an individual to develop a body schema which includes not only a physical image of oneself, but also an assessment of self-worth in relationship to others in the world/social context. The intention of any form of therapeutic use of touch and the attitude of the therapist may therefore contribute to informing and possibly revising the body schema. Therapists using touch in the form of reflexology may not consciously be working within a psychodynamic contract, but the effect on self-image is likely to have some potency and subsequent health benefits.

The nurturing presence of another can elicit responses in an individual, which can be interpreted as being cared for. John Bowlby's early work in the late 1940s focused on the effects of children's early separation from their mothers, evolving a theory of attachment. Bowlby's system of attachment also included the propensity to learn to trust attachment figures from the experience of being supported when distressed. Later, Bowlby proposed guidance on how the attachment theory could be utilised in therapeutic work with clients across the lifespan (Ainsworth & Bowlby 1991). Within any therapeutic relationship, attachment issues can arise, although recognition and analysis of these aspects are more likely within psychotherapy discourse than the practices of touch therapies such as reflexology. The presence of the therapist has been defined in the literature as 'being with' the client in the most fully human, authentic, unique, and open way as possible (Gold 1996). Empathy is felt when the patient becomes aware of the therapist's openness to understanding their situation. A useful way of viewing this is to see it as 'witnessing' how another presents him- or herself, to remain compassionate, curious and open. The process of being witnessed is two-way – clients may be observing therapists for an acknowledgement of his or her understanding through non-verbal responses, elicited from posture, facial expression, respiration and paralinguistic components of speech (Moursand & Erskine 2004; Yardley-Jones 2006).

Reflexology is not a form of psychotherapy or counselling, yet the client can be nurtured by it as part of his or her processing of past or current emotional trauma and distress. Nowhere is this more apparent than for patients experiencing the existential crisis of life-threatening disease, such as cancer. Garnett (2003) conducted semi-structured interviews (informed by feminist interviewing techniques) with 18 therapists from 16 hospices providing reflexology massage and aromatherapy. The thematic analysis of the transcripts led to three observations of the impact and role of touch therapies:

• Complementary therapies facilitating an emotional inoculation
• Sustaining a protective cocoon
• Provided by professional caretakers at a time of vulnerability.

Meeting an individual in such circumstances can result in the person becoming quiet, reflective and tearful. Some clients may be much more expressive, which may be the result of suppressing their emotions for some time. Emotional release can often be accompanied by physical events: release of endorphin-rich tears, changes in breathing patterns (deep and sighing expirations) and changes to the ANS, initially sympathetic arousal and then profound relaxation (parasympathetic) with reduction in blood pressure and heart rate, audible intestinal peristalsis and salivation (Pennebaker 1992; Kettles 1994; Carroll 2002). In reviewing the literature and the definition of the term 'healing crisis' as it relates to reflexology, Mackereth (1999) identified that it can include various physical and emotional responses following, or even during, treatment. The conclusion reached from this review was that patients were probably experiencing and expressing a much-needed emotional catharsis, with permission to unburden, triggered by the potency of the therapeutic space, the touch and attention of a skilled and supportive therapist.

REFLEXOLOGY: PROVIDING A SPACE TO TALK

Trousdall's (1997) study of a series of reflexology for a group of women with mental health problems arose from their negative experiences of mental health care and the reliance on prescribed medication. Following a series of reflexology treatments they were encouraged to make a number of lifestyle changes. As with other studies, the provision of touch and a supportive space in which to share experiences and concerns was acknowledged. In another study, Gambles et al. (2002) used semi-structured questionnaires to uncover the 'existential' benefits of a series of six reflexology treatments given to a total of 34 patients receiving palliative care. The participants reported on the value of time spent talking with a therapist, a typical comment was:

> ... being able to discuss my illness with caring and friendly staff, ... I had so much on my mind – I just talked which was also very helpful [name of the reflexologist] was so very helpful and caring ... she not only made my feet comfy and my mind more calm, but she helped with advice (p. 41).

Gambles (2002) did not report whether the therapists were nurses or lay therapists. The need to talk to 'someone' who can comfort and be helpful clearly can make a difference to a patient's experience of healthcare. A pilot study (n=6) was conducted by Boyd et al. (2001) in which mental health service users reported key sessional themes noted by the reflexologist, including health and social concerns, physical/preventative health strategies and experiences of the health service. Semi-structured interviews with the clients identified recurrent themes, notably their health improvements related to the reflexology, a sense of relaxation, increased interest in self-care, a feeling of being cared for, time for self and reactions with areas treated on the feet. It was suggested that many of the conversations were 'far more meaningful and detailed' precisely because talking was incidental to the intervention.

Practitioners may, or may not, exhibit cues that indicate openness to disclosures; blocking or discouraging, disclosures is a well-recognised phenomenon in healthcare (Booth et al. 1996, 1999). Some patients may disclose information when directly questioned, but others choose to do so when a healthcare professional is performing a physical procedure such as taking the blood pressure or drawing a blood sample, although others will express their concerns unprompted. Greater familiarity with the healthcare professional and greater severity of patients' psychological distress increased the likelihood of disclosures which occurred most frequently during history taking, physical examination and discussion of treatment options (Robinson & Roter 1999).

In a recent randomised, controlled reflexology trial, 50 participants living with multiple sclerosis (MS) were recruited, each receiving six weekly sessions of reflexology delivered by nurse-reflexologists (Mackereth et al. 2009a). Analysis of audio-taped transcripts revealed that women's disclosures were highest during the first and second reflexology sessions, whilst men's disclosures more frequently occurred later, typically in the third or fourth session (Mackereth et al. 2009b). This may be due to the fact that women are more likely to attend voluntarily for reflexology, whereas men are more likely to have been encouraged by partners to attend, or are referred by health professionals. Some clients, particularly men, may need the relationship to have become established before feeling safe enough to unburden themselves. From the available transcripts it appears that some disclosures were made spontaneously by patients, whilst others were triggered by the therapist making direct enquiries related to the reflexology intervention. Therapists also enquired about the patient's well-being without reference to reflexology, sometimes related to a prior disclosure. Therapists also acknowledged disclosures and offered advice on occasions. Crucial to explorations about the role of reflexology in the therapeutic relationship there were numerous examples of 'reflexology-related enquiry' leading to disclosures of worries and concerns.

An example of reflexology-related enquiry is given below (the disclosures are underlined in the text);

Patient (P). That's a bit sensitive, what's that?

Therapist (T). That's the bladder area.

P. I have felt for months now that I don't have the bladder control that I did have. When I want to go to the toilet I have to go immediately, which is very annoying (58G2: 1 F).

In the following extract the transcript included a therapist enquiry, unrelated to reflexology, which resulted in series of disclosures of current concerns; this was picked up again later in the transcript:

T. How is your MS?

P. I take sleeping tablets … one of my problems, a problem with MS … is like fire in my hands, you rub it and it won't go away; the tablets help … then I can't sleep. Heat is a problem it affects the MS [description of a social event in a very warm room] … I had to crawl away (10G2: 1 M).

This study on MS and reflexology included the use of a number of psychological and physiological outcome measures, collected pre- and post-individual reflexology sessions, as a baseline, at the first session and after the sixth session. Whilst there were limitations to the study, significant changes in both anxiety levels and salivary cortisol measurements were identified. The author concluded that reflexology appears to have an effect on stress and well-being, which could be linked to the provision of a space for the disclosure of worries and concerns, as well as the support, advice and positive use of touch (Mackereth et al. 2009a).

PLACEBO AND NOCEBO EFFECTS: EXPECTATIONS AND THE HEALING CRISIS

In exploring the psychological basis for reflexology there has to be an exploration of the view that reported benefits of complementary therapies, such as reflexology, are just placebo effects. Placebo, as a concept, is often simplistically viewed as pleasing the patient, with outcomes being attributed to how the intervention is perceived by the patient (Beecher 1955). Expectation is argued to be a major component of placebo with signals suggesting potency (Crow et al. 1999). For example much work has been done on the components of the placebo effect within pharmacological research, for example the colour of a pill and what is said by the person who prescribes it (Kienle & Kiene 1997). Some drugs, which have clinical effects within a laboratory setting for a certain condition, may have reported effects on another condition even though there is no explanation for this. Any investigative work involving observation, monitoring and gathering of data may influence the behaviour of those being monitored. This is known as the Hawthorne effect, which was originally recognised following time and motion studies in factories.

A concept which is less often discussed but which shares the same perceptual origins as placebo is that of the *nocebo* effect. Here, adverse effects, with characteristics similar to the side effects of specific drugs, are anticipated and experienced by patients, even when a pharmacologically inactive substance, or a substance with no record of the reported side effect is given (Ernst 2001). An example of nocebo, potentially at its most harmful, is that of the 'ritual' of 'informed' consent (Loftus & Fries 2008), whereby practitioners feel obliged to give a detailed list of side effects of treatments, without awareness of how powerful this could be, or without an evidence base for the purported effects. Anxious and trusting patients will then anticipate that they will experience these harmful side effects. For reflexologists, listing possible signs of the so-called 'healing crisis' may be so strongly suggestive that the patient/client will actually experience these symptoms. The picture is clouded by advising clients to drink more water (to eliminate toxins), whilst also claiming that they will pass more urine following a reflexology treatment. In reviewing the available literature, there is no evidence to suggest that these lists of 'detoxi-fication' symptoms result directly from the reflexology treatment. Emotional responses are not uncommon and may have physical consequences, yet these reactions are argued not to be the direct physical effects of the reflexology. Loftus and Fries (2008) postulate that health professionals should engage in conversation about placebo and nocebo when eliciting 'informed' consent, and should encourage patients to be optimistic about side effects. In terms of reflexology, linking physical changes associated with emotional release could be proffered as a helpful process. Our role is to provide support by listening and asking how we can help, for example holding the feet or encouraging the client to curl up on his or her side and providing a comforting cushion or blanket. Using such terms as 'detoxification' may be unhelpful and may serve to pathologise, rather than normalise, the emotional and physical responses (see Case Study 2.1).

CASE STUDY 2.1

Ruth, a carer, was offered reflexology while visiting her partner in the hospice. She responded by saying, 'so long as it's not like the treatment I had on holiday'. Ruth said, 'I was told by this therapist that I would feel very tired, have a headache and pass lots of urine after treatment. Half-way through the one-hour session I was beginning to relax and started thinking about my partner and began to cry. The therapist just kept her head down and did not talk to me, and then worked my feet so hard they hurt. At the end she just said "drink lots of water". That night I slept badly, had a headache and was up and down to the toilet ... she was right – I was exhausted.'

The hospice therapist said, 'It's a positive thing to release emotion. You can express your feelings here. I am here to support you. Indeed, release of emotion will be helpful to you. The touch will be very gentle and if you want me to stop at any time just raise your hand ... you don't even need to speak.' Fifteen minutes into the treatment Ruth did indeed cry and was encouraged to lie on her side with a 'cuddle pillow' while the reflexologist listened to what she said about her partner, and just held her feet. Ruth then drifted off to sleep. After 20 minutes she awoke more refreshed. Ruth returned for weekly treatments and reported sleeping better and having more energy to care for her partner.

The psychological basis for therapeutic outcomes of reflexology

We should not assume that all responses, immediate or delayed, are due directly to the interventions provided. In considering reflexology or any other therapy, a client is making a choice to engage with his or her body and another person's dedicated skills, time and attention. Clients make either conscious or unconscious choices to engage with and express or contain emotion. Expressing emotions is one thing; understanding their origins is another matter entirely. Insight takes reflection and analysis, possibly even professional help through counselling or psychotherapy (see Ch. 5). A reflexologist needs to be wary of blaming himself or herself or the therapy when emotion surfaces. It is better to remain curious and open than to make a judgement about what may or may not have been the trigger(s). Even if you think the intervention or your presence played a role, it is important to acknowledge that you are a compassionate helper whose treatment may have enabled another to engage with his or her feelings and their too-often denied body (Cawthorn 2006). It is important to be professional and accountable for your practice, to have appropriate attitudes and sensitive responses to emotional disclosure. Part of being compassionate and present in therapeutic work is to recognise the honour of witnessing another who is expressing emotional vulnerability.

Understanding the dynamic processes that are part of building rapport and maintaining healthy attachment within therapeutic relationships requires training, knowledge and the ability and motivation to refine interpersonal skills. Boundaries of practice are based upon establishing a contract with clients, clarifying shared therapeutic goals, reflecting on behaviour, intention and content of communication, verbally, written in leaflets and non-verbally in our physical demeanour. Not all of these issues and implications for training have been covered adequately within many traditional practitioner courses. Indeed many of the complex nuances of clinical practice are often not considered until incidents arise and force therapists to revisit their knowledge and skills base. The professional practice of clinical reflexology in healthcare settings requires continuing professional development, maintaining a reflective process on and about practice and ideally engaging in mentoring and/or supervision.

CONCLUSION

Clinical reflexologists need to avoid making claims to cure illnesses; rather, they need to investigate how their work can impact on improving health, maximising well-being and managing symptoms where underlying disease exists. In this chapter, we have explored the route to achieve changes in health via reducing anxiety, improving mood and empowering clients to make lifestyle changes. Reflexology can provide a space for psychological support and nurturing of the body, which in turn helps to influence long-term health and well-being. Additionally, there is evidence in the literature that a series of treatments provides opportunities for deepening the therapeutic relationship and providing a space for conditioning the stress–immune responses. Cumulative benefits can be accrued, strengthening the person's sense of self-worth and building resilience emotionally and physically. In conclusion, it is argued that physiological changes can be a consequence of psychological processes and, given the complexity of the reflexology package, these are likely to be working in synergy (Table 2.1).

The psychological basis for therapeutic outcomes of reflexology

Table 2.1 *The reflexology package – psychological processes and implications for practice*

Factor	Potential for change	Possible outcome	Suggestions for practice
1. Placebo	Expectations of 'health' enhancing benefits	Experiences benefits	Engage with clients about the concepts of placebo and nocebo
2. Nocebo	Listing symptoms of 'Healing Crisis' or 'Detoxification' can lead to expectation of those side effects	Experiences side-effects	Be aware of the impact of language Maintain up to date knowledge of research findings rather than myth
Therapeutic use of touch and contact	'Being with' through physical holding Being met and nurtured at a time of vulnerability, stress and anxiety Potential for creating a therapeutic cocoon (Garnett 2003)	Feel safe and cared for Experience acceptance Empowering experience Able to unburden and disclose	Contract for touch - ability to say 'yes', 'no' or 'stop' Review acceptability of pressure, pace and length of treatment Acknowledge the power of human contact
Cumulative engagement	Emergence of a therapeutic relationship over time Attachment and evolving sense of safety and comfort	Potential muddle about type of relationship and intimacy Disclosure of major life incidents or narrative Client uses the evolving supportive relationship to make lifestyle and other changes	Ensure clarity of professional relationship Review therapeutic goals and expectations of the work and relationship Process of change owned by the client not the therapist Role of mentoring, supervision and ongoing education to assist role development

(Continued)

Table 2.1 *The reflexology package – psychological processes and implications for practice—cont'd*

Factor	Potential for change	Possible outcome	Suggestions for practice
The reflexology map	A curious body schema that engages the client and therapist	Potential for *reflexology-related enquiry* and disclosures (Mackereth 2009b)	Map to be viewed as a territory/landscape for exploration not for diagnosis
Psychoneuroimmunology (PNI)	The links between the emotional state, disease processes and experience – with a two-way relationship between the immune system and the central nervous system (Rabin et al. 1989; Lloyd 1990)	Reflexology package' assists in release of endorphins, reduction in cortisol and other stress hormones	Ensure treatments promotes wellbeing and relaxation Explore with clients how reflexology may help to maintain and improve well-being Maintain and develop knowledge about the psychological and physiological effects of reflexology

Ader, R., 1982. Behaviorally conditioned immunosuppression and murine systemic lupus erythematosus. Science 215, 1534–1536.

Ader, R., Cohen, M., 1975. Behaviorally conditioned immunosuppression. Psychosom. Med. 37, 333–340.

Ainsworth, M., Bowlby, J., 1991. An ethological approach to personality development. Am. Psychol. 46, 331–341.

Beecher, H.K., 1955. The powerful placebo. JAMA 159, 1602–1606.

Booth, K., Maguire, P.M., Butterworth, T., Hillier, V.F., 1996. Perceived professional support and the use of blocking behaviours by hospice nurses. J. Adv. Nurs. 24, 522–527.

Booth, K.M., Maguire, P., Hillier, V.F., 1999. Measurement of communication skills in cancer care: myth or reality? J. Adv. Nurs. 30 (5), 1073–1079.

Boyd, D., Evans, C., Drennan, V., 2001. Using reflexology: a feasibility study. Ment. Health Nurs. 21 (6), 4–16.

Cameron, R., 2002. Subtle bodywork. In: Staunton, T. (Ed.), Body psychotherapy. Brunner-Routledge, Hove.

Carroll, R., 2002. Biodynamic massage in psychotherapy: reintegrating, re-owning and re-associating through the body. In: Staunton, T. (Ed.), Body psychotherapy. Brunner-Routledge, Hove.

Carter, C.S., 1998. Neuroendocrine perspectives on social attachment and love. Psychoneuroendocrinology 23 (8), 779–818.

Cawthorn, A., 2006. Denying the body. In: Mackereth, P., Carter, A. (Eds.), Massage and bodywork: adapting therapies for cancer care. Churchill Livingstone, London.

Conti, F., Pittoni, V., Sacerdote, P., Priori, R., Meroni, P.L., Valesini, G., 1998. Decreased immunoreactive-endorphin in mononuclear leucocytes from patients with chronic fatigue syndrome. Clin. Exp. Rheumatol. 16, 729–732.

Crow, Gage, H., Hampson, S., Hart, J., Kimber, A., Thomas, H., 1999. The role of expectancies in the placebo effect and their use in the delivery of health care: a systematic review. Health Technol. Assess. 3 (3).

DoH FIM NHS Alliance NAPC, 2000. Complementary medicine: information pack for primary care groups. DoH FIM NHS Alliance NAPC.

Dryden, S., Holden, S., Mackereth, P., 1999. 'Just the ticket'; the findings of a pilot complementary therapy service (Part 11). Complement. Ther. Nurs. Midwifery 5, 15–18.

Ernst, E., 2001. Towards a scientific understanding of placebo effects. In: Peters, D. (Ed.), Understanding the placebo effect in complementary medicine: theory, practice and research. Churchill Livingstone, London.

Freud, S., 1923. The ego and the id. SE 19, 3–66.

Gambles, M., Crooke, M., Wilkinson, S., 2002. Evaluation of a hospice based reflexology service: a qualitative audit of patient perceptions. Eur. J. Oncol. Nurs. 6 (1), 37–44.

Garnett, M., 2003. Sustaining the cocoon: the emotional inoculation produced by complementary therapies in palliative care. Eur. J. Cancer Care 12, 129–136.

Gold, J.R., 1996. Key concepts in psychotherapy integration. Plenum, New York.

Jessop, D.S., 2002. Neuropeptides: modulators of immune responses in health and disease. In: Clow, A., Hucklebridge, F. (Eds.), Neurobiology of the immune system. Academic Press: an imprint of Elsevier Science, London.

Kettles, A., 1994. Catharsis: an investigation of its meaning and nature. J. Adv. Nurs. 20, 368–376.

Kienle, G.S., Kiene, H., 1997. The powerful placebo effect: fact or fiction? J. Clin. Epidemiol. 50 (12), 1311–1318.

Lloyd, R., 1990. Possible mechanisms of psychoneuroimmunological interactions. In: Ornstein, R., Swencionis, C. (Eds.), The healing brain. Guildford Press, London.

Loftus, E.F., Fries, J.F., 2008. The potential perils of informed consent. McGill J. Med. 11 (2), 217–218.

Mackereth, P., 1999. An introduction to catharsis and the healing crisis in reflexology. Complement. Ther. Nurs. Midwifery 5, 67–74.

Mackereth, P., Booth, K., Hillier, V., Caress, A., 2009. Reflexology and relaxation training for people with MS: a controlled trial. Complement. Ther. Clin. Pract. 15, 14–21.

Mackereth, P., Booth, K., Hillier, V., Caress, A., 2009. What do people talk about during reflexology? Analysis of worries and concerns expressed during sessions for patients with multiple sclerosis. Complement. Ther. Clin. Pract. 15, 85–90.

Montagu, A., 1971. Touching: the human significance of the skin. Columbia University Press, Columbia.

Moursand, J.P., Erskine, R.G., 2004. Integrative psychotherapy. Thomson, London.

O'Hara, C., 2002. Challenging the 'rules' of reflexology. In: Mackereth, P., Tiran, M. (Eds.), Clinical reflexology: a guide for health professionals. Elsevier Science, London.

Pennebaker, J., 1992. Confiding traumatic experiences and health. In: Fisher, S., Reason, J. (Eds.), Handbook of life stress, cognition and health. John Wiley & Sons, Chichester.

Rabin, B.S., Cohen, S., Ganguli, R., Lysele, D.T., Cunnick, J.E., 1989. Bidirectional interaction between the central nervous system and the immune system. Crit. Rev. Immunol. 9, 279–312.

Robinson, J.W., Roter, D.L., 1999. Psychosocial problem disclosure by primary care patients. Soc. Sci. Med. 48 (10), 1353–1362.

Sutherland, V.J., Cooper, C.L., 1995. Understanding stress: a psychological perspective for health professionals. Chapman & Hall, London.

Tiran, D., 2009. Reflexology in pregnancy: a definitive guide for healthcare professionals. Elsevier, Edinburgh.

Trousdall, P., 1997. Reflexology meets emotional needs. Int. J. Altern. Complement. Med. 9–12 November.

Wall, M., Wheeler, S., 1996. Benefits of the placebo effect in the therapeutic relationship. Complement. Ther. Nurs. 2 (6), 160–163.

Yardley-Jones, T., 2006. The heart and positive emotion – from concept to measurement. J. Holist. Healthcare 3 (3), 5–9.

FURTHER RESOURCES/READING

Hucklebridge, F., Clow, A., 2002. Neuroimmune relationship in perspective. In: Clow, A., Hucklebridge, F. (Eds.), Neurobiology of the immune system. Academic Press: an imprint of Elsevier Science, London.

Mackereth, P., Carter, A. (Eds.), 2006. Massage and bodywork: adapting therapies for cancer care. Churchill Livingstone, London.

Peters, D. (Ed.), 2004. Understanding the placebo effect in complementary medicine: theory, practice and research. Churchill Livingstone, London.

Selye, H., 1974. Stress without distress. Signet, New York.

Educational developments

3

Beverly Newbury • Peter Mackereth

ABSTRACT

Over the last decade we have seen an increased interest in developing educational provision for reflexologists, particularly reflected in the number of academic courses offered within higher education institutions. There has also been a growing demand for courses that promote integration of clinical reflexology within conventional healthcare settings. These and other educational- and practice-related routes enhance therapeutic skills and equip practitioners with the skills required to promote and engage in research.

Academic study requires utilisation of relevant literature: reflexology-specific papers and well-referenced contemporary textbooks; these continue to increase in number and improve in quality. Additionally, texts are available on specialist healthcare fields (e.g. oncology, midwifery and mental health) which feature contributions on reflexology and other therapies. In addition, the staging of a series of national and international reflexology conferences continues to raise the profile of the profession.

This chapter examines key developmental issues in the provision of educational courses, the importance of continuing education and the need for mentoring and supervision of ongoing practice.

There are numerous accounts dealing with historical evidence, principles and practices that are considered to have been instrumental in the development of contemporary reflexology practice. The work of early 'modern' pioneers is also frequently detailed, and the development of early

© 2011 Elsevier Ltd. All rights reserved.
DOI: 10.1016/B978-0-7020-3167-0.00003-2

UK reflexology education is covered in more detail in the first edition of this publication. This chapter will review recent and current preparatory and continuing education provision in the UK and factors that influence the development of professional reflexology skills.

KEY WORDS

Preparatory education, core curriculum, conformity, clinical skills, continuing education, continual professional development (CPD), teaching, safeguarding public, profession, levels of provision, skills progression, supervision.

RECENT AND CURRENT DEVELOPMENTS

Reflexology education and training provision has continued to improve over the past few years from what was once described as a 'cottage industry' (Cant & Sharma 1996), and the reflexology profession is continually seeking to produce skilled practitioners able to operate in a wide 'practice arena'. Achieving this goal is the primary concern of the Reflexology Forum, currently recognised as the developing regulatory (voluntary) body for reflexology in the UK. Through ongoing work, the Forum has helped the profession to 'agree a set of common standards for the practice and training of reflexology' and to 'develop a core curriculum' (Reflexology Forum 2005). The Education and Training Working Group, tasked with the production of the core curriculum, identified disparity in accepted standards of training, echoing previously identified 'disparate provision' (Mills & Budd 2000; Reflexology Forum 2001). With its development being supported by the Prince's Foundation for Integrated Health (FIH) and involving representatives from each of the Forum's professional member organisations, from FIH and Skills for Health, this disparity was addressed through the resulting publication of the 'Core Curriculum for Reflexology in the United Kingdom' in July 2006. The core curriculum provides recommendations primarily aimed at complete preparatory education and training of reflexology practitioners, although some guidance for continual professional development (CPD) is also offered. Curriculum content is mapped against National Occupational Standards initially published by Healthwork UK, now Skills for Health (SfH) (2002), and contains SfH assessment guidelines (Reflexology Forum 2006; Box 3.1; Box 3.2).

BOX 3.1 Core curriculum aims

'This core curriculum brings to the training of reflexology in the UK a common foundation which will end the current disparity in course content and depth. It will provide a thread of continuity between practitioners that could be recognised by, and thus reassure, the general public. The publication of a core curriculum will contribute to the safety and effectiveness of graduates and will provide a standard of learning and skill upon which the rich variety and diversity of the individual practitioner can then be built.' (Reflexology Forum 2006)

BOX 3.2 Clinical skills
Clinical skills term refers to ability to: 'apply safe and effective reflexology techniques to a broad range of clients and adapt these treatments to a wide range of clinical conditions with which clients may present ... minimum curriculum intended to produce practitioners who can work with clinical conditions' 'equally as well with people who seek help for clinical conditions as those who desire a relaxing treatment.' (Reflexology Forum 2006:95)

As training providers conform, delivering courses of sufficient 'content and depth' to meet the quality and standards of the core curriculum, this should eventually lead to all reflexology practitioners having a single identity based on the same core clinical skills (Box 3.1). These skills should form the basis of all reflexology training courses, enabling practitioners to adapt treatments safely and effectively, according to the needs of clients with clinical conditions or clients merely seeking relaxation (Reflexology Forum 2006; Box 3.2).

Reflexology practitioners have a responsibility to engage in personal and continuing professional development (Reflexology Forum 2005; Box 3.3). Many UK reflexologists complete vocational training, provided largely by the private sector and further education colleges, which may be approved by one or more of the professional reflexology bodies. These organisations usually have a designated education officer or panel, application process and assessment procedures. Commonly, a fee is required for the approval process and inspection. Additionally, some form of annual review as a means of quality assurance is standard practice.

A variety of progression routes including academic and professional CPD options enable practitioners to build on knowledge and skills acquired through initial therapy training to develop further theoretical and practice-related skills. Academic routes enable development of analytical and research skills and CPD options can help equip practitioners with skills in specialist areas, for example in cancer or pregnancy care (QAA 2008).

Opportunities to access educational courses within complementary medicine are now widely available, but economic and political factors have recently seen a decline in the number of courses available in higher education institutions. However, practitioners may seek further clinical training to secure employment in healthcare settings. To achieve this, they may choose to combine a series of CPD courses, broader academic study and self-directed work experience/placements.

Continual personal and professional development is also important for teachers of reflexology who have a responsibility to maintain and develop their educational and mentoring skills, and, through continuous and current practice, their clinical skills. Relevant bodies within both professions (reflexology and teaching) also require evidence of CPD in order to maintain membership. Teaching and mentoring standards and provision may vary across training providers; however, the core curriculum (Reflexology Forum 2006) provides clear recommendations for sourcing new teachers of reflexology. In addition to teaching and assessor/verifier qualifications, teachers should produce evidence of

> ## BOX 3.3 CPD practitioner responsibilities
>
> 'Although this curriculum is complete in the education and training of a Reflexology Practitioner, graduates have a responsibility to continually develop their profession (CPD), refine their skill and update their knowledge.' (Reflexology Forum 2006:13)

substantial and current practice experience. Unsupervised course tutors/course leaders should have either 5 years or 1000 hours of continuous and current experience as a reflexology practitioner and supervised course tutors/facilitators should have either 3 years or 600 hours of continuous and current experience as a reflexology practitioner. The curriculum clarifies the importance of practice, stating that 'current, ongoing experience is as important as a teaching qualification' (Reflexology Forum 2006:100). It is worth remembering, however, that although years of experience are invaluable, not all experienced practitioners possess the skills required to become good teachers.

As reflexology is not statutorily regulated, there is no protection of title; therefore, unscrupulous individuals can offer reflexology for monetary gain with little or no training. Some may be self-taught whilst others may have completed an adult education course intended as a 'taster' or for non-commercial use with family and friends. Commonly, they are unlikely to have had any external assessment or monitoring of their skills and are equally unlikely to be members of a recognised professional body. Additionally, they are likely to put patients/clients at risk by not obtaining appropriate insurance. Evidence of professional indemnity insurance can reassure the public, as many insurers require evidence of qualification from organisations that

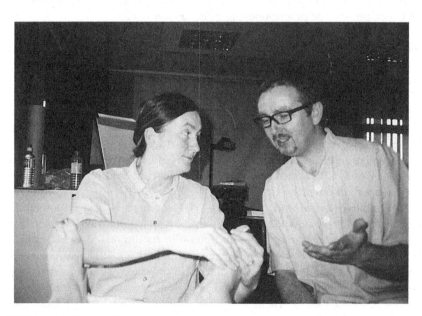

FIG. 3.1 Clinical practice being supervised. *Reproduced from Mackereth P. Journal of Complementary Therapies in Nursing and Midwifery 1999; 5(3):68.*

they consider to provide a reputable standard of education. Unfortunately, inadequately trained individuals may sometimes obtain insurance based on having been awarded a certificate of qualification, which in the past may have been obtained, for example, after attending a two-day course or completing a correspondence course, and which have been accepted by some insurance companies as sufficient evidence of competence to practice.

To protect and safeguard the public and practitioners the profession is working to help in the move to provide independent information through the establishment of a single national practitioner register. This would help to dispel some of the current confusion amongst the public, providing them with an easily accessible source of appropriately trained practitioners (Reflexology Forum 2005). The use of professional registers within the healthcare professions is also supported by the government, and registers are currently being developed as part of voluntary regulation by the General Regulatory Council for Complementary Therapies supported by the Reflexology Forum, and the Complementary and Natural Healthcare Council (HMSO 2007; CNHC 2008; GRCCT 2009). Although there are two alternative options for membership, a register contributes to meeting the government recommendations of regulating the profession 'under a single professional body' (House of Lords 2000; Department of Health 2001). As sufficient evidence of professional status is required to be listed on these registers, reflexologists will seek to maintain and reinforce links with their professional bodies in order to continue their professional development. This will also serve to encourage all prospective and practicing reflexologists to join the many responsible individual practitioners who currently examine their skills and practice to identify any areas requiring attention, which may include consolidating or expanding preparatory education or continuing education and training.

REFLEXOLOGY PROGRAMMES IN THE UK: DIFFERENT LEVELS OF PROVISION

Current educational providers of reflexology training have been divided into three main groups: colleges of further education, the private sector and higher education. These groups offer different levels or bands of training and education. Skills acquired vary according to individual courses, and outcomes may not always reflect claims or meet expectations. Course choices, therefore, ought to be considered carefully.

COLLEGES OF FURTHER EDUCATION

A large number of therapists are trained at colleges of further education, which offer mainly vocational courses (with a qualification) using awarding bodies such as VTCT, ITEC, Edexcel and, more recently, City and Guilds. The qualification or diploma awarded following completion of this type of course is provided at vocational level 3. Some colleges also offer introductory and non-vocational courses (without a qualification). In the early developments of therapy training, provision in colleges often originated through hairdressing and beauty therapy departments and was often linked to beauty therapy courses. Increasingly, therapies have been brought under the banner of 'complementary therapy' or 'holistic therapy' and most colleges now generally offer 'stand-alone' courses, although content and standard of training vary. Course origins and links with beauty therapy have led some to identify this level or band of training as 'salon reflexology', considering that 'beauty level' sounded disparaging to the high skill level attained by many beauty therapists. The term 'salon', however, could also be viewed as downgrading and the profession has not yet agreed on the use of a satisfactory term.

Emphasis in training should be about quality and standards rather than primarily about where the training takes place. Adoption of the core curriculum by training providers across all sectors could eventually eliminate the need for identifying different levels of preparatory training, as all practitioner course providers seek to deliver a common minimum standard of training for learners. If time scales restrict the ability to offer therapy options within larger courses, it may be appropriate only to offer clearly identifiable introductory modules within courses aimed at other professions. Ultimately this would also result in the eradication of inadequate short courses (Reflexology Forum 2006; Box 3.1).

College courses are funded by the Further Education Funding Council (FEFC) and in order to be financially viable often work with large class sizes, sometimes exceeding 20 students. Allocation of course hours can vary considerably from 20 (10 sessions × 2) hours to 108 (36 × 3) hours, which could significantly influence course content and quality. This allocation is often influenced by cost implications, which vary within institutions and across sectors of provision. There are further implications for students studying multiple disciplines as, although courses usually include supervised and assessed client work, limited time allocation can result in newly qualified practitioners lacking confidence to treat the public. The core curriculum makes clear recommendations (Box 3.4).

An attractive feature of further education college courses is that they are often structured to offer more flexible study hours including part-time and/or evening study options. This, combined with the significantly lower student fees compared with the private and higher education sectors, may well influence many students, including health professionals.

THE PRIVATE SECTOR

Private training schools and colleges offer a wide range of preparatory and continuing educational courses in reflexology. Many are linked to professional reflexology organisations, although some are not and training standards vary.

BOX 3.4 Allocation of course hours

The recommendations of the core curriculum are that reflexology training includes 180 teacher contact hours over a minimum of one academic year acknowledging that many training providers across all sectors now run programmes over two years, which should provide students with sufficient time to develop the necessary skills and confidence to become effective practitioners. (Reflexology Forum 2006)

Many private schools and colleges have been started by reflexologists of many years of practice experience, who originate from, or have been influenced by, different reflexology 'pioneers'. The reflexology techniques and underlying philosophy taught, therefore, may differ according to the background of the school. Some schools offer a level or band of training similar to further education college courses termed 'salon reflexology' whist others offer practitioner-level training, which would more suitably be described as 'clinical reflexology' (Box 3.2). Allocation of course hours can also vary amongst courses offered within the private sector, again often influenced by cost implications, although teacher–student ratios can be improved in comparison to most further education colleges, with lower student numbers within study groups. As in any other sector, however, practitioner training courses need to be of an appropriate length and duration in order to meet the requirements of the core curriculum (Box 3.4). Many private schools and colleges have established good local reputations, are accessible and provide good postgraduate support, features which can be crucial in attracting students. The private sector is also able to offer a wide variety of CPD courses serving to provide opportunities for practitioners to access relevant continuing education training suited to their specific needs and interests. Many of these are accredited by one of the reflexology organisations which offer practice credibility, and a few are now credit-rated by the higher education sector, which ensures an acceptable and standardised academic credibility.

UNIVERSITY AND HIGHER EDUCATION

University undergraduate academic level and above (degree level) reflexology modules have increased in availability over the last few years, particularly as new degree programmes in complementary medicine have emerged. Although academic courses have been available at various universities since the first such course at the University of Salford, which commenced in the late 1990s, well-established academic courses specifically in reflexology are rare. The first academically accredited UK reflexology course (1991) ran for a short time at the University of Manchester and was also originally approved by a national educational body for Nursing and Midwifery (Faltermeyer 1995). Reflexology modules are usually incorporated into complementary medicine degrees, although the main focus of these degrees varies across the country. Some programmes do not offer a practitioner qualification; therefore, graduates with no previous professional reflexology qualification would be required to complete an additional course recognised by a registered body in order to practice reflexology. A few private organisations have taken steps to seek academic recognition for their reflexology CPD courses, such as the pregnancy reflexology course offered by Expectancy and credit-rated by the University of Greenwich. The recent introduction of numerous therapy-based foundation degrees may particularly appeal to those who would not have considered the more traditional degree route alternative. Often, these programmes are more accessible, usually available in colleges, which may be perceived by some to be a less intimidating environment. They often offer more realistic study timetables suited to working students, are completed in two to three years and increasingly include practitioner training. For those who already possess appropriate academic and research skills, there are further progression opportunities to achieve top-up degrees, masters' degrees and doctorates (UCAS 2008).

The increased interest in teaching complementary therapies is evident in UK universities and HE institutions and provides timely opportunities for the development of personal and professional skills. Degree programmes have an important role to play in helping students to develop academic abilities at a study level not generally available through other sectors of provision. Students can widen their knowledge, enhancing current skills through critical analysis and evaluation. Research skills can be acquired which equip practitioners to contribute to the future development and advancement of the profession by 'extending the frontier of knowledge' (QAA 2008). This skill base can help to answer increasing calls for further scientific research within complementary therapies (House of Lords 2000; Department of Health 2001). Significantly valuable research has been published by a graduate of the first academic reflexology programme in the UK (Mackereth et al. 2009) and other graduates have published in international peer-reviewed journals on the topic of reflexology (Dryden et al. 1999; Tipping & Mackereth 2000). Another attraction of universities and higher education institutions is that they are able to provide students with a wide range of relevant literature through extensive library facilities including access to interlibrary loans. Many colleges of further education may be able to offer similar facilities; however, private schools often do not have resources of this extent.

Many practitioner courses across all sectors incorporate relevant analysis of the subject built into the curriculum and follow the minimum duration guidelines of one academic year. They may include acceptable assessment strategies of continual practical assessments, case studies and either a written final assessment or examination or a minimum-word assignment (Reflexology Forum 2006). Although levels of monitoring vary across sectors and some schools have minimal provisions in place, many institutions and schools are monitored by internal assessors and moderators and external assessors or examiners. Further education colleges follow procedures inspected and regulated by Ofsted (2008), whilst academic institutions follow Quality Assurance Agency for Higher Education (QAA) and FHEQ guidelines for maintaining academic standards and quality assessment. These agencies coordinate their activities where institutions cross over in their provision (QAA 2008). University-appointed external examiners are usually confined to review of academic assessments; however, attendance at examination boards and production of annual reports contribute to rigor in both managing and providing courses. Additionally, academic institutions are also subject to reviews of their teaching and research activities. External assessment through professional bodies across all sectors is likely to involve observation of clinical assessments and/or moderating written assessments and examination papers. However, a small number of colleges do not work with professional reflexology organisations although they may still review the work of their schools and teachers. Both existing and new programmes need to be developed and designed effectively to meet the ongoing requirements of the profession, adapting content to conform to the core curriculum and to changes which occur within the profession. The theoretical content of more traditionally practical-based vocational courses may need to develop to reflect the depth of the core curriculum; however, critical examination of research evidence, ethical issues and therapeutic models would be more appropriate as development of academic skills at degree level.

Degree courses which do not include practitioner training could be in danger of compartmentalising the practice from the theory of complementary healthcare and need to consider the benefits of integrating theory and practice.

YOUR REFLEXOLOGY CAREER

In summary, when choosing reflexology training and continuing education it is important to consider your specific requirements and expectations as a reflexologist. It is important to establish what level of training is appropriate and to examine course structure and content to ensure that identified needs will be met satisfactorily for your current and future role. In seeking opportunities for personal and professional development beyond preparatory education, it can be useful to develop an action or progression plan to help make choices best suited to both short- and longer-term continuing education and professional development goals. Professional reflexology organisations are usually able to offer advice or guidance and, if accessible, previous graduates can be useful sources for recommendations. We would also advise consulting with coordinators of complementary therapy services and specialist practitioners in conventional healthcare settings (potential employers) about your educational needs, validation of prior experience and appropriate recognised qualifications. Once armed with this information, you may wish to approach and review accessible and acceptable education provision.

It is particularly important for healthcare professionals to examine carefully what is offered in terms of registration and level of practice. Plans to develop reflexology practice within existing healthcare employment would need to involve clinical management in the decision process to ensure that training is also suited to their particular requirements. Producing and following a checklist would be advantageous to anyone when choosing a training course (Box 3.5).

Within higher education provision, there are national systems of accreditation which provide descriptors to illustrate the development of student skills as they progress through different academic levels of education. Modules of learning are credit and level rated which accumulate and progress towards

---

BOX 3.5 Checklist for choosing a reflexology course

- Level of training – preparatory or continuing (CPD – personal and professional)
- Duration of course/hours allocated (see Box 2.4)
- Teacher(s) qualifications and experience
- Structure and content (complying with core curriculum)
- Assessment strategy and academic level (appropriate to personal needs)
- Progression routes available (if applicable)
- Approval and validating bodies, such as universities, colleges and professional reflexology organisations (including appropriate qualification if vocational)
- Quality of teaching packages, handouts and training manuals
- Access to clinical placements and practice clients
- Educational resources, such as library facilities, internet access, teaching environment
- Amount of supervision and tutorial support

Educational developments

BOX 3.6 FHEQ and SEEC – education levels and skills progression

Level 3: FE level 3/HE level 0 – (college certificates)

Limited knowledge/awareness – learning to use cognitive skills to make informed judgements – applying in simple and familiar contexts (with guidance) – applying practical techniques in predictable, defined contexts – limited autonomy (under direction/supervision)

Level 4: HE level I – (higher national certificates and certificates of higher education)

Factual/conceptual knowledge – able to collect and categorise ideas/information and to evaluate – applying accurately to problems beginning to appreciate complexity of issues (with guidance) – applying practical techniques in predictable, defined contexts – limited autonomy (under direction/supervision)

Level 5: HE level 2 – (foundation degrees, diplomas of higher education and higher national diplomas)

Detailed knowledge/awareness of wider implications – able to compare and reformat ideas, evaluate with relevance/significance – identify key elements of problems and choose appropriate methods for resolution (with minimum guidance) – applying practical techniques in complex and unpredictable situations – increasing autonomy (reduced supervision/direction)

Level 6: HE level 3 – (university degrees (honours) and graduate certificates and diplomas)

Comprehensive knowledge/awareness of personal/professional responsibilities – able to transform concepts, critically evaluate evidence – applying knowledge and skills to complex problems – applying practical techniques in complex and unpredictable contexts – autonomously (minimal supervision/direction)

(SEEC 2003; QAA 2008)

---

the final award. These can also be achieved through independent study, prior learning, experience, research and portfolio development which, once assessed, can attract transferable or accumulated credits/points. Box 3.6 details relevant levels and associated development of skills from further education vocational level 3 to academic degree level 6. Expectations include increasing depth of 'knowledge and understanding', developing complexity of cognitive abilities (analysis, synthesis, evaluation and application) and attaining increasing autonomy in the application of 'practical skills'.

CONCLUSION

It is essential that all preparatory education courses across all sectors of provision cover the same minimum standard of training. These must conform to the requirements of the reflexology core curriculum to ensure parity of educational provision. This will ensure that all graduates have studied sufficient content and depth over a specified time period to assimilate and develop in all aspects of their education (Box 3.1; Box 3.4) enabling them to acquire sufficient theoretical and clinical practice skills to become competent, confident, autonomous practitioners (Box 3.2). Practitioners also have the responsibility to engage in personal and professional development through continuing education to help maintain and develop professional skills with the added benefits of gaining specialist skills and maximising their potential as well as contributing to the development of the profession. Links with professional bodies are essential as they provide support mechanisms for graduates to access throughout their professional practice. This important element, together with time and experience, will enable graduates to make the shift from competent to confident practitioner.

REFERENCES

Cant, S.L., Sharma, U., 1996. Professionalization of complementary medicine in the United Kingdom. Complement. Ther. Med. 4, 157–162.

CNHC – Complementary and Natural Healthcare Council, 2008. On-line. Available: www.cnhc.org.uk/pages/index.cfm; 1 June 2009.

Department of Health, 2001. Government Response to the House of Lords Select Committee on Science and Technology's Report on Complementary and Alternative Medicine. HMSO, London.

Dryden, S.L., Holden, S.D., Mackereth, P., 1999. 'Just the ticket': the findings of a pilot complementary therapy service (part II). Complement. Ther. Nurs. Midwifery 5 (1), 15–18.

Faltermeyer, T.S., 1995. Working towards quality – developing an approved course. Complement. Ther. Nursing Midwifery 1 (5), 138–142.

GRCCT – General Regulatory Council for Complementary Therapies, 2009. The UK Federal Regulator for Complementary Therapies. On-line. Available: www.grcct.org/; 1 June 2009.

HMSO, 2007. Trust, Assurance and Safety – The Regulation of Health Professions in the 21st Century – Government White Paper. HMSO, London.

House of Lords, 2000. Select Committee on Science and Technology. Sixth Report on Complementary and Alternative Medicine. HMSO, London.

Mackereth, P.A., Booth, K., Hillier, V., Caress, A., 2009. Reflexology and progressive muscle relaxation training for people with multiple sclerosis: a crossover trial. Complement. Ther. Clin. Pract. 15, 14–21.

Mills, S., Budd, S., 2000. Professional organisation of complementary and alternative medicine in the United Kingdom 2000. Centre for the Complementary Health Studies. University of Exeter, Exeter.

Ofsted. About us – Services we inspect or regulate, 2008. On-line. Available: www.ofsted.gov.uk/Ofsted-home/About-us/Services-we-inspect-or-regulate; 1 June 2009.

QAA – Quality Assurance Agency for Higher Education, 2008. The framework for higher education qualifications in England, Wales and Northern Ireland (FHEQ), second ed. Quality Assurance Agency for Higher Education, Gloucester.

Reflexology Forum, 2001. The EaT Report on reflexology education and training in the UK. Reflexology Forum, Manchester.

Reflexology Forum, 2005. About us – what is the Reflexology Forum. On-line. Available: www.reflexologyforum.org/aboutus.htm; 1 June 2009.

Reflexology Forum, O'Hara, C.S. (Ed.), 2006. Core curriculum for reflexology in the United Kingdom. Douglas Barry, London, 13, 95, 100 & cover.

SEEC Southern England Consortium for Credit Accumulation and Transfer, 2003. Credit Level Descriptors for Further and Higher Education. SEEC, Essex.

Skills for Health – National Occupational Standards for Reflexology, 2002. Competence application tools. On-line. Available: www.tools.skillsforhealth.org.uk/; 1 June 2009.

Tipping, E., Mackereth, P., 2000. A concept analysis: the effect of reflexology on homeostasis to establish and maintain lactation. Complement. Ther. Nurs. Midwifery 6 (4), 189–198.

UCAS, 2008. Courses starting in 2009. On-line. Available www.search.ucas.com; 1 June 2009.

Educational developments

USEFUL RESOURCES

Centre for Clinical Reflexology, Email: admin@clinical-reflexology.org. Website: www.clinical-reflexology.org.

Clinical Association of Reflexologists (CAR) (formerly known as Centre for Reflexology) Denby House Business Centre, Taylor Lane, Loscoe, Derbyshire, DE75 7TA

Expectancy Ltd, Expectancy offers professionally and academically accredited continuing professional development courses for reflexologists, on pregnancy, childbirth, infertility and women's health, www.expectancy.co.uk.

Reflexology Forum, The Reflexology Forum, Dalton House, 60 Windsor Avenue, London, SW19 2RR, Telephone: 0800 037 0130. Email: admin@reflexologyforum.org. Website: www.reflexologyforum.org.

Ethical, legal and professional principles

4

Julie Stone

CHAPTER CONTENTS

ABSTRACT

Whilst few reflexologists are likely to be sued in the course of their professional practice, all practitioners owe their patients a duty of care and must work within the law. Ethical, legal and professional responsibilities are integral to safe and effective practice. This chapter will outline the major ethical and legal responsibilities owed by reflexologists to their patients.

KEY WORDS

Benefiting, not harming, confidentiality, consent, ethical, legal duty of care, limits of competence, respect for autonomy.

INTRODUCTION

Although there has been growing awareness of the therapeutic potential of reflexology, the ethical and legal issues facing practitioners have received little specific attention, perhaps because of the assumption, on the part of

DOI: 10.1016/B978-0-7020-3167-0.00004-4

both practitioners and patients, that reflexology is gentle and non-invasive, and therefore harmless. Nevertheless, any therapy that has the capacity to benefit a patient also has the capacity to cause harm, for example, when used inappropriately, or counter-therapeutically, or where a practitioner exceeds the bounds of his or her competence (Stone 2002). As reflexology becomes more professionalised, therapists must start thinking more about their ethical, legal and professional responsibilities. Issues such as seeking consent to treatment, respecting a patient's confidentiality, and maintaining appropriate boundaries are relevant to all healthcare professionals, including reflexologists. Greater awareness of the issues protects both clients and practitioners, and cultivation of high ethical standards, together with an enhanced evidence base, will help reflexology to be regarded as a mature, reflective profession.

ETHICAL AND LEGAL DUTIES TO BENEFIT AND NOT HARM PATIENTS

BENEFICENCE AND NON-MALEFICENCE

Patients are entitled to expect that their therapeutic encounter with a reflexologist will provide benefit in the form of symptomatic relief or enhanced well-being. So too, patients are entitled to expect that their encounter with a reflexologist will not cause them harm. These expectations (reflected in law as rights) are encapsulated in the ethical duties of beneficence (benefiting) and non-maleficence (not harming) – ethical principles that are at the heart of all healthcare relationships. The therapeutic relationship is a 'fiduciary' relationship, whereby patients trust practitioners with access to their personal information and permit close touch, trusting that the reflexologist will be motivated, at all times, by the patient's interests. These duties form the basis of reflexology codes of ethics and are a central plank of Western and non-Western healing traditions (Stone 2002). As in most complementary and alternative (CAM) therapies, the notion of what constitutes 'benefiting' in reflexology is somewhat wider than within conventional medicine. Whereas medical benefit usually involves the removal of symptoms, reflexology may benefit patients by preventing illness from arising or may improve the patient's mental outlook on his or her condition through relaxation. Equally, however, the notion of harm is somewhat broader, and can include not just physically injuring a patient, but also causing emotional harm, or preventing the patient from seeking more appropriate treatment. Therapists must always avoid making inappropriate claims for reflexology, and indeed are bound by the laws pertaining to specific conditions, for example, not guaranteeing to cure cancer, not providing maternity care except in an emergency and not attempting to treat sexually transmitted disease.

SCOPE OF PRACTICE AND LIMITS OF COMPETENCE

To be able to benefit patients, reflexologists must be competent. Competence requires both technical proficiency, including keeping up to date with advances in research and clinical practice, and ethical literacy. This means the ability to analyse and reflect upon ethical dilemmas arising in practice. As many reflexologists work single-handedly in private practice, therapists must recognise their own limits of competence and should be willing to refer on where necessary, either to a more experienced reflexologist, or to another CAM practitioner, or to a medical doctor, as appropriate. Whilst holistic therapists can, conceptually, offer some level of benefit to all patients, practitioners must be realistic about not treating patients, or not continuing to treat patients, for whom little benefit is likely.

'Best practice' demands not just high standards of pre-registration training, but also a commitment on the part of the reflexologist, once qualified, for continuing professional development (CPD) and, where possible, supervision of practice (Mackereth 2001). In the statutory health sector, CPD is increasingly regarded as a requirement to remain on a professional register, and it is likely that CAM professions will adopt this principle too. Reflexologists should also keep themselves up to date with current research in order that practice can be based on the best available evidence. Whilst individual practitioners may not wish to become research active, they should nonetheless undertake audit of their practice to ensure that they are delivering consistent and acceptable outcomes.

Increasingly, codes of ethics now stipulate that reflexologists must themselves be in good physical and mental health in order to be able to treat patients effectively and safely. Working as part of a multidisciplinary team, or being in receipt of supervision, may help an individual to acknowledge a period where it is not prudent to practice. Failure to do so may result in a fitness-to-practice hearing and removal from a professional register.

REFLEXOLOGISTS' DUTY OF CARE

The ethical duty to benefit patients is mirrored by a legal and professional duty of care requiring practitioners to treat patients with all due care and skill. Reflexologists who fall short of their duty of care and cause patients harm may be found negligent if sued in a civil court, or they might have to face a fitness-to-practice hearing before a professional body. Patients are more likely to resort to legal action when they are unable to seek redress through any other means. Negligence may arise out of any sphere of a reflexologist's activities, such as failure to diagnose adequately or correctly, negligent treatment or negligent failure to disclose risks to the patient before providing treatment.

Negligence does not require the patient to demonstrate that the reflexologist *intended* to cause the patient harm. In determining whether a reflexologist has been negligent, a court would, broadly speaking, apply the 'Bolam test' of professional negligence. This test derives from the legal case of *Bolam v. Friern Hospital Management Committee* 1957. Although it has been slightly modified by subsequent case law (Hope et al. 2008), its main principle holds good, which is that the standard of care owed by a reflexologist to a patient is that which could be expected of a reasonably skilled and competent reflexologist acting in the given circumstances. Reflexologists must act in accordance with practice which would rightly be accepted as proper by a responsible body of professional opinion. This allows considerable latitude for how reflexologists treat, as it means that practitioners will only be negligent if they act in a way which no reasonable practitioner would have acted. In ascertaining 'reasonableness', the court would look to national standards and professional requirements in place at the time of the incident, such as National Vocational Qualifications, or the standards contained in the CNHC's code of ethical conduct, and/or evidence would be sought from an expert witness. The absence of a single professional standard within reflexology at the time of writing presents difficulty in ascertaining the appropriate standard of reasonableness. Currently, the incidence of litigation against reflexologists arising out of their professional practice is minimal, and this is reflected in the low premiums for personal professional indemnity insurance which are paid by clinical reflexologists. Paradoxically, the rate of litigation may increase as reflexology becomes more popular and visible.

MAINTAINING SAFE, EFFECTIVE BOUNDARIES

Safe, effective therapy requires safe, effective boundaries. Boundaries denote the safe and appropriate limits of professional relationships, based, at all times, on the best interests of the patient. When boundaries are breached, for example by practitioners acting in a sexually inappropriate way, or by practitioners becoming overly reliant on their patients to meet their own emotional or financial needs, this can result in serious and enduring harm to patients. It is always the professional's responsibility to set and maintain clear boundaries (CHRE 2008). Although reflexologists are no more likely to abuse the relationship of trust than any other health professional, allegations of professional abuse have been raised against the range of regulated and unregulated health professions (Halter et al. 2007). Moreover, the particular dynamics and the context of the complementary and alternative medicine (CAM) relationship may increase the likelihood of boundary violation by both therapist and patients. For example, many reflexologists work in sole private practice out of their own homes or visit patients in their homes; they do not work as part of a team, and may not receive any sort of professional supervision. They may treat friends or friends of friends, or others with whom they have a dual relationship, and may actively cultivate a relaxed, 'easy-going' atmosphere, as distinct from a sterile, clinical environment. Each of these factors may exacerbate the risk of unclear boundaries (Stone 2008).

Whilst incidences of deliberate sexual abuse are uncommon (although it is difficult to detect prevalence with any accuracy), it is important to acknowledge that emotional and sexual attraction does occur on the part of practitioners and on the part of patients (Halter et al. 2007). The therapeutic use of touch is particularly potent, and reflexologists must be aware of the risks of using touch with certain clients, cultivating empathy and warmth whilst at the same time setting unmistakable professional boundaries around the context of touch and the professional relationship. Practitioners should be particularly mindful of how their actions may be interpreted by the patient, for example, a regular welcoming or departing hug being misconstrued as a sexual advance. Similarly, overfamiliarity on the part of the reflexologist may cause the patient mistakenly to consider the therapist as a friend. Reflexologists should also be mindful of inappropriate levels of self-disclosure which can be a precursor to breaching boundaries. Entering into business arrangements with patients or their family, and lending and borrowing of money from patients is almost always inappropriate and liable to lead to misunderstanding and bad feeling.

Although it would be regrettable if, in order to prevent these problems, reflexologists felt bound to practice more defensively, practitioners must also be aware of the professional dangers of an allegation of abuse and should take the relevant steps, such as the maintenance of detailed, contemporaneous notes, or the use of chaperones if needed, to avoid unfair or inaccurate allegations being made against them.

REFLEXOLOGISTS WHO COMMIT CRIMES

The criminal law applies to practitioners as it does to any other individual. Whereas negligence involves unintentional harm, successful criminal prosecutions rely on the State (in the form of the Crown Prosecution Service) being able to prove beyond reasonable doubt that a reflexologist both committed a criminal act *and intended to do so*. Examples of criminal offences include sexually assaulting a patient, drug offences, or stealing money from a patient. Falsifying one's tax return, for example by failing to disclose income from patients who paid in cash, would also constitute a criminal offence. Notably, criminal convictions will impact on registration with a professional body, and within the statutory sector, serious criminal convictions often result in removal from the professional register.

One would hope that few, if any, reflexologists would be prosecuted in connection with their professional practice. As well as having dire personal consequences for the practitioner, criminal acts within professional practice would breach the primary ethical principle to do patients no harm. They would also be a breach of the fiduciary relationship that is at the heart of the therapeutic encounter, in which the patient should be able to assume that the reflexologist will act at all times in the patient's best interests.

RESPECTING THE PATIENT'S AUTONOMY

Respecting autonomy means allowing patients to make decisions about their own lives and to act in accordance with their own set of values and preferences. Most reflexologists consider that they provide treatment that is individualised, holistic and ultimately patient-centred. Certainly, one would hope that a therapeutic encounter in which the patient is given the time and space to explore his or her feelings at length, as well as discussion of physical symptoms, would facilitate the patient's involvement in the therapeutic process and increase their sense of empowerment. For reflexology to be maximally efficacious, patients have to be active participants in their own healing, making whatever adjustments to diet, exercise, stress levels or mental outlook the practitioner recommends.

Conversely, this does not mean that reflexologists are incapable of acting paternalistically, such as when practitioners believe that they 'know better' and seek to override the patient's wishes or fail even to elicit the

Ethical, legal and professional principles

patient's views. Such behaviour is considered outmoded within medicine as an abuse of the professional's power and is no more acceptable in clinical reflexology than in other healthcare relationships. In condemning paternalism, we must not, however, lose sight of the fact that some patients might *want* their reflexologist to make some decisions for them. Sometimes, otherwise autonomous patients may luxuriate in allowing themselves to become temporarily dependent upon a therapist for a period of time. Whilst it is imperative to seek consent from a patient who does have mental capacity, absence of capacity does not rule out a therapeutic relationship. Reflexology can provide benefit even when patients are not autonomous (e.g. where they are suffering from learning disabilities or are incompetent minors). In such situations, the practitioner's ethical and legal obligation is to act in the patient's best interests. What is important is that when patients wish to be autonomous reflexologists do not supplant the patients' values and preferences with their own.

ETHICAL REQUIREMENTS OF THE DUTY TO RESPECT AUTONOMY

Most of the ethical requirements to do with autonomy concern the giving of information. To redress the power disequilibrium inherent in the professional relationship, the reflexologist must disclose as much information as the patient needs or desires to know in order to make an informed decision whether or not to enter into or proceed with treatment. This will include information about the therapy, how long each session is going to last, how many sessions are likely to be necessary, what the reflexology is likely to achieve and, if the patient wants to know, information about the reflexologist's training and therapeutic orientation. Practitioners should also discuss what they will expect of patients, for example, being aware of and telling them about any side effects after treatment, being honest and open in giving a history, and paying for missed sessions. Respect for autonomy involves treating the patient as an equal in decision-making and keeping them informed and involved as the therapeutic relationship deepens. Consent, critically, is not a one-off exercise, but an ongoing process, and reflexologists should continue to check with patients that they are happy to proceed with specific interventions and the therapeutic relationship.

Respecting autonomy also requires that the reflexologist treats as confidential any information given by the patient during the therapeutic consultation (including disclosing to third parties the fact that the patient is in receipt of treatment). Patients invariably disclose a significant amount of personal information in the course of their treatment. They do so trusting that this information will be used solely for their benefit. However, reflexologists need to be able to explain to patients that this duty is not absolute and that there may be rare situations when the reflexologist may be obliged to breach the patient's confidentiality (Case Study 4.1).

Reflexologists should familiarise themselves with their professional code of ethics and be aware of the particular circumstances in which strict confidentiality may be overridden. This might include the legal duty on the part of the

Jeanette had been receiving regular reflexology for a few weeks when she confided to her reflexologist that she was pregnant for the second time and that, because of her dissatisfaction with the first experience, she had decided to care for herself during this pregnancy and that her partner was intending to deliver the baby at home without midwifery support. Jeanette did, however, wish to continue to receive reflexology throughout the pregnancy.

The reflexologist felt very concerned about this and discussed the case anonymously with her supervisor, who informed her that it is illegal for anyone other than a midwife or doctor to deliver a baby except in an emergency (see Ch. 10). However, the dilemma for the practitioner was being asked to continue the treatment in the knowledge that Jeanette was pregnant and at risk of complications as a result of her previous delivery. She could not be seen to be colluding with Jeanette's wishes and yet could not break Jeanette's confidentiality by referring her to the local midwifery service, which she had no desire to use.

The practitioner advised Jeanette that she would be willing to provide reflexology care during the pregnancy on condition that Jeanette sought the appropriate maternity support. Jeanette was given contact details of the local Supervisor of Midwives but declined to follow this up, so the reflexologist felt obliged to withdraw her services.

reflexologist to inform the local Medical Officer in the case of discovering that a patient has a notifiable disease or, rarely, if the patient tells the reflexologist something in the course of a treatment session that causes the reflexologist to fear that the life or safety of a third party is at risk. An example might be if the patient confides to the reflexologist that he or she intends to commit a serious assault on a named individual, and the reflexologist genuinely believes that breaching confidentiality and warning the individual will significantly reduce the likelihood of that individual suffering harm.

LEGAL FACETS OF THE DUTY TO RESPECT AUTONOMY

The law may protect a patient's autonomy in a number of ways. The civil action of battery directly protects a patient's bodily autonomy. A battery occurs if a reflexologist touches a patient, for example, in the course of a physical examination, without having obtained consent. In most therapeutic situations, a patient's consent to be touched may be implied if the patient lies down and makes no obvious objection to examination or treatment. Consent can only be implied to things that a reflexologist could be reasonably certain that the patient would agree to if asked directly, and good practice demands that consent is explicitly sought, and recorded in the patient's notes. The concept of implied consent would not permit, for example, a vaginal or rectal examination as part of a physical examination, which, in any case, would be wholly inappropriate within standard reflexology practice, although it may be relevant if the therapy was incorporated into midwifery or gynaecological nursing practice, and agreed as part of a protocol with the nurse or midwife's employing organisation.

The second legal action arising out of autonomy and information giving is an action for negligence for failing to provide appropriate information. A hypothetical example might be a reflexologist failing to warn a diabetic patient about the risks of treatment, if the patient underwent treatment unaware of those risks, and suffered harm caused by the reflexology. However, this extends only so far as contemporary evidence available at the time.

Reflexologists are also under a legal, professional and ethical duty to respect confidentiality. Occasionally, a patient might be able to sue a reflexologist who disclosed confidential information learned in the course of the professional relationship, particularly if economic loss was sustained as a result of the unauthorised disclosure. Reflexologists must also comply with their ethical legal responsibilities in relation to data protection, and ensure that their manual and computer records are maintained in accordance with statutory requirements. Data protection legislation extends a practitioner's duty to safeguard certain manual as well as computer-based health records. Although reflexologists are not yet included in the list of professionals who are duty-bound to allow their patients access to their records by law, they should do this as a mark of respect for autonomy, and might even wish to consider providing patients with a copy of their records.

JUSTICE, FAIRNESS AND GOVERNANCE REQUIREMENTS

Principles of equality, justice and fairness are an important aspect of ethical practice. As service providers, reflexologists are obligated to comply with laws and regulations ensuring that all patients are treated equally irrespective of gender, disability, sexual orientation, or age (except where differential treatment is therapeutically indicated). Many of these ethical and legal requirements are also contained within reflexologists' codes of ethics, which require practitioners to treat all patients fairly and with dignity.

PROFESSION-WIDE AND INDIVIDUAL REGULATION

The current common law allows freedom to practice, by which anybody can set up as a reflexologist (or other complementary therapist) with limited training, or indeed, no training whatsoever. This degree of variation places a high degree of trust on individual practitioners to act ethically and in the best interest of their patients. The proliferation of regulatory bodies makes it hard for patients to choose a competent therapist, other than by word of mouth, and renders it difficult for commissioners (e.g. the NHS or third-party insurers) to contract with therapists. Currently, in the UK, a reflexologist may belong to one of a number of professional registers. Prospective patients should be encouraged by the practitioner to contact his or her professional organisations to confirm minimum training requirements and qualifications. The professional body should also be able to provide information regarding their code of ethics, which will determine the standard of professional behaviour expected of its therapists, as well as any complaints mechanisms that exist in the event of something going wrong in the course of treatment.

The previous regulatory diversity has rendered it hard to achieve profession-wide standards setting or standardisation. This situation is now improving as reflexology has recently come under the auspices of a new umbrella voluntary register within CAM, the Complementary and Natural Healthcare Council (CNHC). Established by the Foundation for Integrated Health, and set up with funding support of the UK Department of Health, the CNHC is well positioned to become a central source of self-regulation for a number of therapies, including massage therapy, nutrition and aromatherapy (see http://www.cnhcregister.org.uk/).

MEETING GOVERNANCE REQUIREMENTS

Whereas reflexologists working within the NHS may have to adhere to NHS governance requirements as part of their contractual terms and conditions of service, independent practitioners need to take their own responsibility for ensuring that basic governance requirements are in place, which requires reflecting on their practice and having systems for ensuring continuous quality improvement (Wilkinson et al. 2004). Independent practitioners need to be aware of risks in their practice and practice environment, and to mitigate against these, for example by providing patients with standardised forms of what reflexology is about, what a treatment session is likely to involve, what the risks and side effects of reflexology are, and what the contraindications to treatment are. It is not possible to predict all risks which can occur in practice, but good governance requires practitioners to think proactively about risks and how to reduce these so far as possible. This includes having protocols in place for when things go wrong, and a visible complaints process including the name of any regulatory body to whom the patient can make a complaint if they feel unable to raise the issue with the practitioner.

RESPONDING WELL TO COMPLAINTS

Responding appropriately to complaints is an important ethical requirement. Evidence shows that complaints which are mishandled by practitioners are more likely to escalate, and may result in complaints to professional bodies, and can result in litigation or the threat of litigation. Although many reflexologists work as sole private practitioners, they should nonetheless adopt the principles of good complaints handling which now apply in health and social care (Dept of Health 2009).

As part of good governance, reflexologists should have a clear and accessible complaints process, and should facilitate patient complaints rather than dismiss them. Rather than acting defensively when a patient complains, reflexologists should regard this as an opportunity to learn from what has gone wrong, and a practitioner should always attempt to resolve any complaint promptly and to the client's satisfaction. As providing redress is an integral part of any complaints system, practitioners should be prepared, where appropriate, to apologise for their actions, and, if need be, refund any fees. Whilst mistakes do sometimes happen, patients are less likely to complain if they understand fully what the risks of reflexology are and have been warned about any possible side effects. Reflexologists should also

Ethical, legal and professional principles

scrupulously avoid creating unrealistic expectations, e.g. as to cure, or speed within which symptoms may be improved, as these are another likely source of complaints.

CONCLUSION

Reflexology is generally thought of as safe and non-invasive, and it may mistakenly be assumed that few ethical and legal issues arise. The purpose of this chapter has been to demonstrate that ethical and legal issues arise in all professional relationships and that the harm that an incompetent reflexologist may cause a patient need not be physical. The requirements of ethical and legal principles go beyond requiring that the reflexologist be technically competent. For clinical reflexology to continue to grow in credibility as an adjunct to mainstream healthcare, practitioners must be familiar with their ethical and legal responsibilities and accept that they are accountable to their patients, their profession and to society as a whole. As well as fulfilling individual responsibilities, reflexologists should take responsibility for the collective aspects of their profession, volunteering, for example, to participate in the profession's disciplinary mechanisms and mentoring colleagues who have recently qualified. Hopefully, adherence to the principles outlined above will ensure that reflexology continues to grow in reputation, respectability and credibility and that adverse incidents remain few and far between.

REFERENCES

Bolam v. Friern Hospital Management Committee, 1957. 1WLR 582.

Council for Healthcare Regulatory Excellence, 2008. Clear sexual boundaries between healthcare professionals and patients: responsibilities of healthcare professionals. CHRE.

Department of Health, 2009. Listening, responding, improving: a guide to better customer care. http://www.dh.gov. uk/prod_consum_dh/groups/dh_ digitalassets/documents/digitalasset/ dh_095439.pdf (accessed 2 September 2009).

Halter, M., Brown, H., Stone, J., 2007. Sexual boundary violations by health professionals – an overview of the published empirical literature. Council for Healthcare Regulatory Excellence.

Hope, T., Savalescu, J., Hendrick, J., 2008. Medical ethics and the law. The core curriculum. second ed. Churchill Livingstone, London.

Mackereth, P., 2001. Clinical supervision. In: Rankin-Box, D. (Ed.), The nurses' handbook of complementary therapies, second ed. Baillière Tindall, London, pp. 33–42.

Stone, J., 2002. An ethical framework for complementary and alternative therapists. Routledge, London.

Stone, J., 2008. Respecting professional boundaries. What CAM practitioners need to know. Complement. Ther. Clin. Pract. 14, 2–7.

Wilkinson, J., Peters, D., Donaldson, J., 2004. Clinical governance for complementary and alternative medicine. Project Report. University of Westminster, London.

FURTHER READING

Cohen, M., Kemper, K., 2005. Complementary therapies in pediatrics: a legal perspective. Pediatrics 115 (3), 774–780. doi:10.1542/peds.2004–1093. http://pediatrics.aappublications.org/cgi/content/full/115/3/774 (accessed 19 September 2009).

Heller, T., Lee-Treweek, G., Katz, J., Stone, J., Spurr, S. (Eds.), 2005. Perspectives on complementary and alternative medicine. Open University Press and Routledge, London.

Hope, T., Savalescu, J., Hendrick, J., 2008. Medical ethics and the law. The core curriculum, second ed. Churchill Livingstone, London.

Lee-Treweek, G., Heller, T., MacQueen, H., Stone, J., Spurr, S. (Eds.), 2005. Complementary and alternative medicine: structures and safeguards. Open University Press and Routledge, London.

USEFUL RESOURCES

For Bioethics resources, see: http://www.unc.edu/cell/files/bioethics/links.html.

Introduction to the UK legal and judiciary system, http://www.direct.gov.uk/en/CrimeJusticeAndTheLaw/Thejudicialsystem/DG_4003097.

Ethical, legal and professional principles

Reflection in reflexology practice through the use of narrative

5

Christopher Johns

CHAPTER CONTENTS

ABSTRACT

This chapter explores the potential for reflection and reflective practice to aid learning and enhance practice. It particularly focuses on the use of narrative, which can be a useful aid to facilitate the therapist to develop sensitivity and to learn from experience. Narrative involves describing in writing a recent experience in practice, then using a formal framework to reflect on it, exploring feelings, emotions, and practical and other issues which may assist in improving, changing or affirming practice for the future.

KEY WORDS

Reflection, reflective practice, narrative, model for structured reflection.

INTRODUCTION

In order to progress with their professional practice, clinical reflexologists need to develop the skills of reflection. Reflection is the process of learning through everyday experiences, enabling us to gain insight towards our

DOI: 10.1016/B978-0-7020-3167-0.00005-8

practice. Through reflection we learn to become cognisant of the factors which constrain us, those which are either embodied within ourselves or embedded within normal organisational patterns. Through that understanding we can then act to shift them so that our visions can be realised, and, as such, reflection can be described as action-orientated. Reflection is an advanced skill which can be refined as time goes on, but one which has become vital in contemporary practice, providing the rationale behind our actions and words and stimulating our sensitivities to patients/clients, their treatments, their health or illness and their psychosocial well-being.

The reflective practitioner is curious about his or her practice and experiences with clients/patients, always challenging his own feelings, thoughts and actions. He or she is not attached to patterns of thinking and responding but is always open to new ideas, always open to learning. The practitioner maintains a commitment to find the 'best way' to practice, knowing that the clients deserve nothing less. The intent of the reflexology practitioner is, perhaps, to touch and thereby to ease the client's suffering in a way which is best for that individual. Yet suffering has an intangible quality which is not easily grasped: it is sensed by, rather than known to, the therapist who needs to be sensitive enough to feel its nature. Knowing how best to respond is a focus of reflective inquiry. Responses can never be taken for granted simply because each situation is unique, even though it may be similar to other previous experiences – but it is not *this* experience. The reflective practitioner is mindful, approaching each situation as if a mystery is unfolding. Who is this person? What meaning does this person give to their experience? 'Meaning' changes like the tides in the roller-coaster of ill-health, particularly within the author's own field of working with people with terminal illness.

NARRATIVE TO AID REFLECTION

Reflective practice can be facilitated through the use of a written narrative and a systematic process of inquiry based on the content of the narrative (Johns 2002).

There are six dialogical movements to the process of reflective narrative:

1. Dialogue with oneself to write a rich, descriptive story of a particular experience that pays attention to detail involving all the senses (*story text*);
2. Dialogue with the story text as an objective and disciplined process (using a model of reflection) to gain insights (*reflective text*);
3. Dialogue between the *text* and other sources of knowing in order to frame emerging, tentative ideas from the text within the wider community of knowing;
4. Dialogue between the text's author and a guide/mentor to clarify, deepen and co-create insights;
5. Dialogue within the hermeneutic spiral to weave the coherent and reflexive narrative that adequately plots the transformative journey (*narrative text*) (The hermeneutic circle describes the process of understanding a text. One's understanding of the text as a whole is established through reference to the individual parts and vice versa. Neither the whole text nor any individual part can be understood without reference to one another.);

6. Dialogue between the narrative and the narrative readers/listeners towards a consensus of insights (*evolving text*).

As such, the six movements take the narrator (practitioner) through the stages of writing, moving through story text (what you write in your journal), reflective text (your reflection on description), narrative text (the presentation of insights in a coherent and reflexive pattern informed by dialogue with literature and with guides), into an evolving text through dialogue with readers and listeners. It is a systematic process of inquiry (Johns 2009).

Before considering in more detail the steps in this process, it may be helpful to consider the issues inherent in the following narrative about the interaction between Mary and the author.

CASE STUDY 5.1 A REFLECTIVE NARRATIVE

Mary is a young-looking 63-year-old lady who had a mastectomy the previous year for breast cancer, but liver and bone metastases were then diagnosed. She is also diabetic and becomes very nauseous prior to eating. Her greatly enlarged liver is squashing her abdomen, making it difficult for her to breathe and her nausea difficult to manage. Curative options have been ruled out and we are on the long trajectory toward death. She feels its relentless pull and I am told she is anxious, although she appears to bear her tragedy with equanimity. One morning, on entering her room, I immediately detect that she is in pain and rearrange her pillows to ensure she feels more comfortable; she declines a heat pad which she had used during the night. The breakfast tray arrives but Mary's appetite is poor, even though she knows that, being a diabetic, it is important to eat some breakfast. I suggest giving her reflexology later that morning, which may help her appetite before lunch.

It is 11.20 before I am back with Mary and she has been looking forward to the reflexology. I ask her how she feels and she tells me she is nauseous. 'No,' I say, 'how do you *really* feel?' She looks down and says she feels alone, that she knows she is going to die. She tries to be brave with her husband and children but finds it hardest seeing her grandchildren. Her mother died from breast cancer and she fears it is hereditary, but no one talks of these things. That's why she feels so alone, as if some conspiracy of silence surrounds her to avoid upsetting her. I suggest maybe they avoid such issues for their own comfort. Mary can see some truth in that. 'As a family we have always avoided talking about difficult things, Jim, my husband, in particular.' I make a mental note to ask him 'how things are' when he visits that afternoon.

And yet, I am uncertain about pushing such issues. Perhaps I should have said, 'How are things?' in a more casual way rather than so directly and intensely – offering Mary the choice of whether she wanted to look more deeply at herself and her dying – although I know from past experience that people often appreciate the opportunity to go more deeply. Every person is different and such ethical judgement is always tentative, as if feeling my way along the person's wavelength. Perhaps I should have asked Mary if she had spoken of her feeling to others, yet there was no mention of this in her notes. But then 'notes' don't always tell the story. I feel comfortable talking to Mary whilst I give the reflexology treatment and she does not resist me. There is something about complementary therapy that opens an intimate space which fosters trust. I know that this space is vital for giving therapy and hence the preparation. I am not satisfied just to walk into a room, give the reflexology and walk out again. I visit once a week and have come to know Mary well, so should I be so concerned to open an intimate space? Is this more for my benefit than for Mary's? To touch someone with our spirit is healing. Cancer rips through people, through families, tears them apart, fragments them. My intent is to ease suffering, to enable Mary to feel whole again. Reflexology is sacred space (Quinn 1992), where touch is a spiritual encounter, touching Mary's spirit with my own. As such I have to nurture my own spirit. I do not tell Mary this; it is the ground for going deeper. I know that my presence in itself is healing, lifting Mary to a higher level of being (Rael 1993).

Her feet and lower legs are very dry and oedematous and she says they ache constantly. My training as a reflexologist was 'technique' focused – really just working the whole foot three times. Over time I have relinquished the emphasis on technique and learned to listen to the person's body. For me, every therapy is an experiment, an opportunity to deepen my craft. This is why reflection is so vital to gain insight into myself as a therapist to become more effective in my quest to ease suffering. To be a holistic therapist is to appreciate the pattern of the whole person and any symptom against the whole. Hence, as I hold her feet I tune more deeply into her. As I do so I centre myself, bringing myself fully present to the moment. I hold her feet for about 5 minutes with my hands flat against the soles of her feet: a point of stillness in a frantic world. I do not usually pay much attention to various parts of the body, but today I dwell over the reflex zones for her liver and shoulders where the cancer has spread. Her liver reflex zone is pale and soggy. I simply hold the liver reflex point with a corresponding reflex point on the top of her foot. I feel the emptiness of this area, seeking to find an energetic balance. It takes a few minutes and then it pulses in. I repeat this on the other foot.

Just then the door bangs open; her lunch is being delivered. Time has passed too quickly and lunchtime has intruded on our space – or perhaps I have intruded on lunchtime. I whisper, 'Keep it warm; I'll bring it to Mary when we are finished.' I can say that with equanimity, whereas previously I would have been irritated. After the reflexology there is more colour and warmth in the feet and Mary has a sensation of energy running up her legs and has no pain or nausea, but now she does not want to move and does not want her lunch. I offer to return with her lunch in half an hour. Mary reported sleeping extremely well after the reflexology and feeling better in herself. She is due to go home the next day but will return twice a week for reflexology, although I offer her the chance of home visits if travelling becomes too difficult for her.

Let us now consider each of these steps in more detail.

1st MOVEMENT – DESCRIPTION – THE STORY TEXT

Reflective notes should normally be written within 24 hours of the experience. It may be useful to keep a reflective diary for making significant notes which can later be transferred to the narrative. *Rich description* is vital because it opens the mind to pay attention to the situation and the environment, drawing on all the senses (Johns 2009). Consider the narrative above and think about what may be significant.

Reflection is learning through everyday experiences towards gaining insights and helping us to realise our visions of practice as a lived reality. Through reflection we learn to become cognisant of those factors, either embodied within oneself or embedded within normal organisational patterns that constrain us. Being cognisant, we can then act to shift them so that our visions can be realised. As such, reflection is action-orientated.

A model for reflection such as the Model for Structured Reflection (MSR) (Fig. 5.1; Box 5.1) is an invaluable guide to assist you, especially if reflection is a new idea. The MSR consists of a series of sequential cues to enable the therapist to explore the depth and breadth of reflection, essentially moving along a spiral from what is significant about this experience to gaining insight. The spiral represents the idea that these insights are enfolded within us.

It takes care and patience to learn the skill of reflection and how to use narrative, so now re-read the narrative above, this time more carefully and patiently, taking time to scrape the surface of the experience, and read between the lines. What else might be significant or, perhaps, less obvious? And as you delve deeper, more significance emerges, which will, of course, be of relevance to you and to your own practice. Perhaps reading the narrative triggers something which might cause you to think about a recent experience of your own.

The cue 'How was Mary *really* feeling?' opens a pathway to developing empathic inquiry. The cue 'What were the consequences of the practitioner's actions for the patient, others and himself?' is a gateway to developing practical wisdom. Consider what the consequences of the practitioner's actions might be, not just the more obvious short-term consequences but also the potential long-term ones. The cues are very deep and revealing of oneself – so be careful! For example, the cue 'What factors influence the way I am thinking, feeling and responding' is not an easy one to work through, simply because we largely take for granted that we ourselves are normal. As we become more mindful we become more aware of oneself within the moment and the way these factors influence us. The revealing of oneself that emanates from this cue is a reason why guidance, support and clinical supervision can be necessary to help us see ourselves and beyond ourselves. It can expose

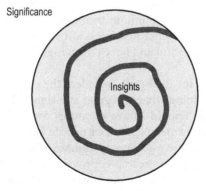

FIG. 5.1 The Model for Structured Reflection.

BOX 5.1 The Model for Structured Reflection (Edition 15ª)

Reflective cue

Bring the mind home

Focus on a description of an experience that seems significant in some way (story/video etc.)

What particular issues seem significant to pay attention to?

How were others feeling and why did they feel that way? (empathy)

How was I feeling and what made me feel that way? (sympathy)

What was I trying to achieve and did I respond effectively?

What were the consequences of my actions on the patient, others and myself?

What factors influence the way I was/am feeling, thinking and responding to this situation?

What knowledge did or might have informed me?

To what extent did I act for the best and in tune with my values?

How does this situation connect with previous experiences?

How might I reframe the situation and respond more effectively given this situation again?

What would be the consequences of alternative actions for the patient, others and myself?

What factors might constrain me responding in new ways?

How do I NOW feel about this experience?

Am I more able to support myself and others better as a consequence?

What insights do I draw from this experience?

Am I more able to realise desirable practice? (framing perspectives)

our vulnerability and the fragility of our coping mechanisms. Reflection is an ontological process of *being* and becoming the reflexologist you need to be, not simply an epistemological issue concerned with *doing* reflexology.

The cue 'What was I trying to achieve and did I respond effectively'? gets to the core of your practice. All action is purposefully geared towards achieving preset aims. Should the practitioner have encouraged Mary to talk about her dying and how was that, or could that be, achieved effectively? These are not easy questions to answer, because at the time, actions taken are those which seemed the right thing to do. As such, judging the effectiveness of one's treatment or actions cannot be truly objective. Did the reflexology improve her appetite? Was the combination of different reflexology techniques the most effective? Every situation is a unique encounter in which there are no immediate solutions to fix problems, just our intuitive sensing within the moment if we are sufficiently mindful and have criteria against which we can measure ourselves.

The cue 'Did I act for the best?' considers the ethical basis for practice – 'the best' – meaning doing what was good and right. This can be approached by posing dilemmas: 'Should I have done this or that?' Such consideration is informed by different perspectives of people and by their informed and ethical principles, including autonomy, utilitarianism, beneficence and non-malevolence (see Ch. 4). For example, do you think that the length of time the practitioner spent with Mary is an ethical issue? Note other ethical issues within the narrative. The cue 'What knowledge did, or could have, informed me?' opens a path to reveal a dialogue with relevant literature to inform practice and help to frame insights. The cue 'What were the consequences of my actions for the patient, others and myself?' is a gateway to developing practical wisdom. Consider what might be the consequences of your actions and everything about your interaction with the client, not just the more obvious short-term consequences but also the possible long-term ones. Use your imagination for, without doubt, actions have consequences.

3rd MOVEMENT – DIALOGUE BETWEEN TENTATIVE INSIGHTS AND THE WIDER FIELD OF KNOWING

Cassell (1991) views suffering as a threat to the other's integrity of wholeness. It is not easily reduced into parts although some authors have tried to reduce it to core dimensions so it can be known and more specifically responded to as if a symptom of terminal illness (Deneault et al. 2004). This author has explored the work of Harrison (2000) and Younger (1995) in his own search for the meaning of suffering in daily practice and within himself (Johns 2006).

The therapeutic claims which a practitioner may make about the value of reflexology could be questioned: the evidence base is not strong, especially when one considers that the particular style of reflexology used by one practitioner may be different from that used in a specific research study. Reflexology is not a controllable variable between therapists. This author uses both vertical and precision reflexology, yet no research was found when preparing this chapter to suggest the efficacy of these approaches beyond anecdotal claims. Reflexology is an intuitive therapy. The ideas of Eckhardt Tolle (2001), O'Donohue (1997) and Jones and Jones (1996) can guide you to explore yourself spiritually and may assist in clarifying ideas, becoming sensitive to nuances and learning from experiences, which can be invaluable for your practice.

Looking back, it is useful to ask oneself, given the situation again, would you respond differently? This cue, perhaps more than any other, helps to focus one's developing insight. It leads from reflection, in which one is looking back at a situation which has already occurred, to anticipating one's actions in future experiences. In doing so, this may plant seeds in your mind which germinate in new situations. So what might you do differently? Perhaps the practitioner in the narrative might have talked to other staff about Mary rather than just reading her notes, but that might have constrained him, or given an impression that may not have been Mary's reality. It raises issues about the scope of the reflexologist's role and the way it fits into the wider caring team.

In this narrative, the timing of the therapy became problematic, as lunch intruded. Mary was sleepy after the treatment and did not want her lunch. Interestingly, her appetite improved slightly over the next two days, but perhaps that was due to better management of her pain and nausea. It is difficult to delineate the benefits of reflexology from other treatments: it may be assumed that her improvement was due to pharmacological responses simply because these responses have been more objectively proven. However, experience dictates that reflexology does have a deeply calming effect on many recipients and, although this remains to be proven conclusively by formal research studies, one cannot dismiss the 'evidence' of personal experience and

Reflection in reflexology practice through the use of narrative observation. The practitioner could, perhaps, have suggested to Mary that she could have reflexology after lunch when her husband would be visiting, which may have opened up avenues for discussion with both of them. On the other hand, the intent of the reflexology treatment before lunch was, superficially, to attempt to improve Mary's appetite. Another change in practice which may occur as a result of the disturbance through the arrival of lunch could be the production of a sign for the door, reading 'Therapy in progress – please do not disturb'.

4th MOVEMENT – GUIDANCE

Reflection is not easy. It requires openness, curiosity, commitment, authenticity and discipline. Perhaps you have clinical supervision where you can share and reflect on such experiences with colleagues. Guidance gives challenge and support but those involved in guiding others need to be skilled at the process, able to stand back enough to pose insightful questions rather than to give answers, who can open the imagination and creativity of their colleagues to explore new, more effective ways of *being* and *doing* in their roles. This takes discipline and perseverance.

5th MOVEMENT – WEAVING THE NARRATIVE

Having written the description, reflected on it using the MSR, explored relevant and diverse literature and talked it through with peers and guides to deepen insight, the narrative can now be written around these newly acquired insights. This can be done by breaking down the original descriptive text into single lines, as if opening the space between the lines where meaning often lies hidden. As you break open the lines, you may find yourself rewriting some of the text, perhaps more poetically to capture particular moments. The underlying intent of writing narrative is to enchant and challenge the reader, to stir their own reflections towards easing suffering and creating better worlds for ourselves and for our patients (Okri 1997). Carefully read again the narrative about Mary. What insights do you perceive? How do these relate to your own practice? You might like to use metaphors, symbols, images, artwork, even dance to capture the deeper meaning. In doing so, narrative moves into *performance*. But then practice itself is a performance. How might you plot your journey of easing suffering, given its intangible nature? There is certainly a sense of easing suffering in the narrative simply through the text. Reflecting on experiences relating to similar events may help to demonstrate how insights gained from one experience inform future events. This is the nature of reflexivity: a looking back to reveal the transformative journey of being and becoming the therapist you desire to be – perhaps more effectively to appreciate and respond to suffering.

6th MOVEMENT – DIALOGUE WITH OTHERS

Using a story (experience) to open a dialogical space enables you to explore stories from your own practice. Within any narrative, it is a question of pulling some aspect out to explore but never losing sight of the whole – what might be described as holistic learning. In doing so, you can deepen your own understandings. It is useful to share your experiences and narrative reflections with other colleagues, who may shed new light on issues you have found difficult to clarify, and who may also feel benefit from the experience of mutual reflection.

CONCLUSION

Through reflection, the reflexologist can become more mindful in their daily practice, almost as if that practice has become an unfolding narrative. If you are permanently centred, you will be mindful of how you are thinking, feeling and responding within the moment, whilst holding the intent to ease suffering and guarding against egoic distraction. Reflection is a valuable tool to learning and to enhance your practice. Whilst it takes time and patience to refine the skills of reflection, it is worth persevering, because deeper understanding and insight of the individual practitioner will ultimately contribute to refinement and progress of the profession of reflexology.

REFERENCES

Cassell, E., 1991. Recognizing suffering. Hastings Cent. Rep. 21 (3), 24–32.

Deneault, S., Lussier, V., Monteau, S., Paille, P., Hudon, E., Dion, D., et al., 2004. The nature of suffering and its relief in the terminally ill: a qualitative study. J. Palliat. Care 20 (1), 7–11.

Harrison, E., 2000. Intolerable human suffering and the role of the ancestor: literary criticism as a means of analysis. J. Adv. Nurs. 32 (3), 689–694.

Johns, C., 2002. Guided reflection: advancing practice, second ed. Blackwell, Oxford.

Johns, C., 2006. Engaging reflection in everyday practice. Blackwell, Oxford.

Johns, C., 2009. Becoming a reflective practitioner, third ed. Wiley-Blackwell, Oxford.

Jones, B., Jones, G., 1996. Earth dance drum. Commune-E-Key, Salt Lake City.

O'Donohue, J., 1997. Anam Cara: spiritual wisdom from the Celtic world. Bantam, London.

Okri, B., 1997. A way of being free. Phoenix House, London.

Quinn, J., 1992. Holding sacred space: the nurse as healing environment. Holist. Nurs. Pract. 6 (4), 26–35.

Rael, J., 1993. Being and vibration. Council Oak Books, Tulsa.

Tolle, E., 2001. The power of NOW. Hodder & Stoughton, London.

Younger, J., 1995. The alienation of the sufferer. Adv. Nurs. Sci. 17 (4), 53–72.

FURTHER READING

Hawkins, P., Shohet, R., 1989. Supervision in the helping professions. Open University Press, Buckingham.

Mackereth, P., 2001. Clinical supervision. In: Rankin-Box, D. (Ed.), The Nurses' Handbook of Complementary Therapies. Churchill Livingstone, London.

Mackereth, P., Carter, A., 2006. Professional and potent practice. In: Mackereth, P., Carter, A. (Eds.), Massage & bodywork: adapting therapies for cancer care. Elsevier Science, London.

Richardson, J., Tate, S., Leonard, O., Paterson, J., 2003. Developing clinical supervision for complementary therapy educators. J. Altern. Complement. Med. 9 (5): 783–787.

Rose, M., Best, D. (Eds.), 2005. Transforming practice through clinical education, professional supervision and mentoring. Elsevier Science, London.

Reflexology: expanding the evidence

Helen Poole • Peter Mackereth

CHAPTER CONTENTS

ABSTRACT

Despite an increase in research into reflexology, evidence for its effectiveness remains limited. This chapter considers the need for research in reflexology and the questions to be asked. We briefly consider research ethics, describe some common research designs with their limitations, and provide an overview of more recent studies and their findings. Both authors have completed PhD studies investigating reflexology; these are briefly summarised along with others reported from 2000 to 2009 (see Table 6.1).

KEY WORDS

Evidence-based practice, methodology, ethics, future developments.

INTRODUCTION

The first edition of *Clinical Reflexology* included a chapter which looked at some of the published research evidence for reflexology. Since then, more studies have been completed, further informing the evidence base for reflexology. It is necessary, first, to consider why research is important to reflexologists as well as the users and service purchasers, and to outline common research methods.

DOI: 10.1016/B978-0-7020-3167-0.00006-8

The Select Committee on Science and Technology (2000) report recommended that well-designed research trials be conducted on touch therapies such as reflexology, which claim to complement orthodox medicine and 'clearly, to comfort' many people. However, the Committee felt that attempts to integrate complementary and alternative medicine (CAM) therapies within UK health services are unlikely to succeed, despite increasing popularity with patients, whilst there remains a paucity of research and lack of practitioner regulation (House of Lords 2000), and 'pump priming' funding for CAM research by the NHS and Medical Research Council was recommended. The report also charged healthcare practitioners (doctors and nurses) with the lead role in advising the public about suitable CAM therapies. To rise to this challenge, the reflexology profession needs to become better regulated, and to produce evidence of safety and effectiveness of a credible calibre to inform healthcare practitioners and enable them, in turn, to advise the public.

Evidence-based medicine, or evidence-based practice, is not new, having evolved to ensure safe and effective care for patients, and is increasingly being adopted in all types of healthcare provision (Sackett et al. 1996). For example, the National Institute for Health and Clinical Excellence (NICE) produce evidence-based guidelines for a range of health technologies (including CAM, pharmaceutical, surgical, psychological and physical therapies) which are used for decision-making about NHS service provision and funding. Reflexologists need to provide evidence for their practice, but other non-reflexologist researchers will also be keen to explore effectiveness and safety of the therapy.

RESEARCH DESIGNS

When considering research, it is necessary to select the most appropriate research design to answer your particular research question. A comprehensive review of all research methodologies is beyond the scope of this chapter. We have chosen, instead, to summarise some of the main types of commonly used research designs and to discuss some of the criticisms of these methods (Table 6.1).

SEEKING USERS' VIEWS

Seeking opinions from users of reflexology via surveys or interviews may provide useful information, but is limited to users only. There are many non-users: people who have not considered reflexology, or who have insufficient information to make a choice, or who lack the financial resources to access private reflexologists. Traditional 'use of reflexology' studies generally focus on positive experiences. For example, Gambles et al. (2002) gathered 'user' perspectives via a semi-structured questionnaire (six items) with a convenience sample of 34 patients attending for between four and six reflexology treatments at a hospice. Patients' feedback was overwhelmingly positive, with accounts of relief from tension and anxiety, feelings of comfort and support from the therapists and improved well-being. Many patients associated the treatment with being better able to cope with their diagnosis and conventional treatment. The hospice staff and therapist distributed the questionnaire, which

Reflexology: expanding the evidence

Table 6.1 Brief summary of research reviewed

Study	Purpose/condition	Method	Treatment/group	Outcome measures	Findings	Commentary
Grealish et al. 2000	To assess the effects of foot massage on nausea, pain and relaxation in hospitalised patients with cancer	Crossover RCT n=87	1. 2 sessions of foot massage, and 2. Quiet resting	HR, Pain (VAS) Nausea (VAS) Self-report of relaxation (VAS)	Significant difference in all measures. Improving relaxation and reducing nausea and pain	No control for medication No exploration of lasting effects Numbers in each group not given. 10 min sessions only. Therapists were trained as reflexologists
Hodgson 2000	To assess the effects of reflexology on quality of life of people in the palliative stage of cancer	Randomised controlled trial n=12	1. Reflexology 2. Foot massage	Quality of Life VAS	2 in foot massage group (6) reported improvements All 6 in reflexology group had significant improvement Verbal reports of satisfaction and benefit	Same practitioner for both interventions. Difficulty with distinguishing between placebo and true reflexology. Small sample. Erroneous omissions of 5 out of 28 components in the VAS scale. No account made of cancer type
Stephenson et al. 2000	To assess the effects of reflexology on pain and anxiety in patients with lung and breast cancer	Quasi-experimental crossover trial n=23	1. Reflexology 2. No intervention period	Pain (SF – MPQ) Anxiety (VAS)	Significant decrease in anxiety following reflexology for both groups. Significant decrease in pain for breast cancer group	Only 2 out of the 10 lung cancer patients reported pain compared to 11 out of 13 in the breast cancer group. Gender difference in the group and effects of pain relief makes it difficult to interpret results

(Continued)

Table 6.1 *Brief summary of research reviewed—cont'd*

Study	Purpose/condition	Method	Treatment/group	Outcome measures	Findings	Commentary
White et al. 2000	Investigation into the accuracy of reflexology charts as a diagnostic tool	Experimental study with 18 patients assessed by 2 practitioners	Assessment time 20 minutes	Comparison of the assessments made by both reflexologists	Ability to distinguish conditions very poor. No evidence of agreement between the practitioners	Assessment time limited to 20 minutes. Not able to communicate to patients. Relied on palpation only. Does not reflect normal reflexology practice. Only 2 practitioners in the study (over 12 000 in UK)
Boyd et al. 2001	Evaluation of reflexology provided to users of a mental health service	Qualitative study n=6	Semi-structured interviews	Thematic analysis of the interview data	Recurrent themes; improvements related to the reflexology, sense of relaxation, interest in self-care & felt cared for/ time for self	Small sample. Practitioner as researcher may have influenced responses
Gambles et al. 2002	An evaluation of a hospice-based reflexology service	Qualitative study n=34	Semi-structure questionnaires	Thematic analysis of the questionnaire data	Positive comments; improved well-being, comfort support, able to cope with symptoms and treatment	Hospice staff and therapist distributed the questionnaire. No demographic details. Sensitive approach taken given the vulnerability of service users in this setting

Smith 2002	Evaluation of reflexology for patients with breast cancer undergoing radiotherapy	Randomised controlled trial n=150	1. Reflexology 2. Foot massage 3. Standard care only	POMS, Pearson-Byars Fatigue Check list, Lymphocyte activity	Significant differences for foot massage compared to standard care group in some subscale of the POMS & Fatigue Checklist. Trend for a possible effect on lymphocyte activity in reflexology group.	Researcher also the practitioner. Used foot massage as a sham treatment
Tovey 2002	Evaluation of the overall effectiveness of reflexology to improve symptoms for people with IBS	Single blind trial n=34	1. Reflexology 2. Foot massage	HADS, 5-point scale: abdominal pain, constipation/diarrhoea, bloatedness, overall health well-being, tiredness	No significant difference between groups with the IBS symptom scale. Significant difference for reduction in anxiety for the reflexology group only	Lead reflexologist advised on the treatment protocol. 6 treatments given as per 'normal practice'. Small study. IBS subtypes not defined
Williamson et al. 2002	To examine the effects of reflexology for menopausal symptoms	Randomised controlled trial n=76	1. Reflexology 2. Sham – foot massage only 3. Maintained usual care	WHQ subscales of Anxiety and Depression, Flushes and night sweats VAS	No significant differences between groups. Small differences favouring reflexology in mean differences for anxiety and depression	MYMOP data invalidated by inconsistencies in its completion. 14 participants reported they knew they were receiving reflexology
Mollart 2003	To explore the effects of two different reflexology techniques versus rest on ankle and foot oedema in late pregnancy	Single blind randomised controlled trial n=55	Reflexology to zones other than lymphatic system (n=20). Reflexology to lymphatic zone (n=25). Rest (n=10)	Ankle and foot circumference measurements. Participant questionnaire (stress, tension, anxiety, foot changes)	No significant differences in foot or ankle circumference between groups. Self-reported well-being statistically improved in lymphatic group and non-lymphatic group compared to rest	Self report to therapists may be biased

(Continued)

Table 6.1 *Brief summary of research reviewed—cont'd*

Study	Purpose/condition	Method	Treatment/group	Outcome measures	Findings	Commentary
Stephenson et al. 2003	To examine duration effects of reflexology in patients with cancer	Randomised, repeated measures experimental study n=36	Foot reflexology × 2 sessions, 2 hours apart No treatment, but offered reflexology session at end of study	Pain scores Medication use (opioids) recorded for 3 consecutive days	In reflexology group, pain scores lower 24 hours after the intervention though not statistically significant. And medication increased	Assistant collected data, not therapist An expectation effect may have occurred in the control group who were promised treatment at the end of the study
McNeill et al. 2006	To investigate the association of antenatal reflexology with different outcomes in the intranatal period	Comparative retrospective cohort design n=150	1. Reflexology (n=50) 2. Control (n=100)	Mode of delivery, Type of onset of labour, duration of labour, use of analgesics	No significant differences in onset or duration of labour between groups Significantly lower use of Entonox in reflexology group	Authors note that standardised treatment and outcome measures would have improved the study quality
Wilkinson et al. 2006	To examine the effects of reflexology for patients with chronic obstructive pulmonary disease	Randomised controlled trial n=20	1. Reflexology 2. Control	Lung function test, evaluation (Quality of Life), HADS, AQ20 Diary Cards BP & HR	No significant changes in lung function, BP & HR No difference between groups on HADS, AQ20, Quality of Life Patients who received reflexology reported feeling better on the evaluation questionnaire	Difference in group characteristics at baseline could have impacted on the results Objective measures showed no differences yet patients self report did. Self report is subject to bias but could indicate patients experienced changes not detected by other measures due to small sample size

Author/year	Aim	Design	Intervention	Measures	Results	Limitations/comments
Quattrin et al. 2006	To examine the effectiveness of reflexology in hospitalised cancer patients during chemotherapy	Randomised controlled trial n=30	1. Reflexology foot massage 2. Control group	STAI	Statistically significant reduction in reflexology group compared to control group	Small sample size. Only measured immediate/next day effects. Treatments provided by student nurses. Patients not categorised by disease
Gunnarsdottir & Jonsdottir 2007	Does the experimental design capture the effects of complementary therapy?: a study using reflexology for patients undergoing coronary artery bypass graft surgery	Randomised controlled experiment n=11	Reflexology Rest	STAI, BP, HR, respiratory rate	No significant differences between groups on STAI, BP, HR, respiratory rate	Small sample size with 2 dropping out of the study. Measures may not have been sensitive to change – participants' comments indicated a change in well-being. The SAI may not be culturally sensitive (Iceland)
McVicar et al. 2007	To explore the effects on reflexology on anxiety, salivary cortisol, melatonin secretion, pulse rate and blood pressure	Randomised controlled trial with crossover design n=30	1. Reflexology 2. Control quiet resting	STAI, BP & HR, salivary cortisol & melatonin	No significant differences between groups on BP, HR, salivary cortisol & melatonin. Significant reduction in state anxiety following reflexology	High drop out rate with only 18 completing the study. Sitting may have been stressful for some individuals
Wyatt et al. 2007	To evaluate patient characteristics to predict selection and maintenance of a complementary therapy	Non-randomised quasi-experiment n=96	Patients could choose 1. Reflexology 2. Guided imagery 3. Guided imagery plus reflexology 4. Interview only	Quality of life Patient characteristics	Those who chose 1, 2, or 3 tended to be older and in worse health with higher anxiety, depression and poorer physical and emotional well-being	Patients without caregivers were restricted to guided imagery or interview

(Continued)

Table 6.1 *Brief summary of research reviewed—cont'd*

Study	Purpose/condition	Method	Treatment/group	Outcome measures	Findings	Commentary
Stephenson et al. 2007	Partner-delivered reflexology effects on cancer pain and anxiety	Randomised controlled trial n=86	1. Partner delivered reflexology 2. Control group	BPI, VAS	Reduction in pain and anxiety in partner-delivered reflexology group	The researcher provided the training and collected the data. Immediate effects could be transient
Poole et al. 2007	Investigation of the effectiveness of reflexology on chronic low back pain	Randomised controlled trial n=243	Reflexology (6 sessions) Relaxation (6 sessions) Usual care (GP)	Sf-36 Pain Oswestry Disability Questionnaire	No significant differences between groups	5 reflexologists provided the treatment Trends in the data showed pain reduction greater in reflexology group
Brown & Lido 2008	To evaluate reflexology as a means of pain relief and empowerment in patients with phantom limb pain	Same subject experiment n=10	Same subjects had 6 sessions of reflexology, followed by 6 sessions of training, then 6 sessions self treatment	Pain diaries, HADS, lifestyle changes	Improvement in phantom limb pain and lifestyle Changes maintained at 12 months follow-up	Lack of control group limits conclusions of this small cohort study

Hodgson & Andersen 2008	To examine the efficacy of reflexology in individuals with mild-to-moderate dementia	Crossover trial n=21	1. 4 weeks of reflexology followed by 4 weeks of friendly visits 2. The reverse	Salivary amylase, Nonverbal Pain checklist, Apparent Affect Rating Scale	Significant reduction in pain and salivary alpha-amylase when receiving reflexology compared to friendly visits	Small sample size. Consent and feedback issues as participants had mild to moderate dementia. Same practitioner did both arms of the study
Quinn et al. 2008	To investigate the effectiveness of reflexology in the management of low back pain	Randomised controlled trial n=15	1. Reflexology group 2. Sham group	Pain VAS, Roland-Morris disability questionnaire, Sf-36, McGill pain questionnaire	Pain VAS clinically significantly reduced in reflexology group. No other significant differences between groups. Both improved on Roland-Morris, McGill and some SF36 subscales	Small sample size – need larger numbers to draw any definite conclusions. Sham group received foot massage
Mackereth et al. 2009a,b	1. To compare the effects of reflexology and progressive muscle relaxation training for people with MS 2. Analysis of worries and concerns expressed during reflexology	Crossover trial n=50	1. Reflexology 2. Progressive Muscle Relaxation Training (PMR)	1. GHQ 28 SAI SF 36 Salivary cortisol, HR & BP 2. Analysis of audiotaped sessions (n=245 tapes)	1. Only significant difference in state anxiety and cortisol levels favouring reflexology. Significant difference in systolic blood pressure favouring PMR 2. Reflexology created opportunities for disclosure of worries and concerns for 48 participants. Recurring themes identified. Differences noted in the subgroups (sex, disease groups)	1. Evidence of carryover effect from one treatment to the other. Crossover design may not have been appropriate 2. Recordings a crude method of eliciting process/content of the sessions. Unbalanced number in the disease subgroups

(Continued)

Table 6.1 *Brief summary of research reviewed—cont'd*

Study	Purpose/condition	Method	Treatment/group	Outcome measures	Findings	Commentary
Woodward et al. 2009 (in press)	To evaluate the effectiveness of reflexology in treating idiopathic constipation in women	Prospective single group test and retest trial n = 19	Reflexology (6 sessions – 45 minutes each)	Gut transit markers & X-ray, Bowel diary, HADS, SF-36 HCAMQ	Improved colon transit times Significant positive change in attitudes towards CAM Improvements in HADS & 3 of the Sf-36 subscales (vitality, general and mental health) Reports of improvement in constipation for most participants (94%)	Small study. No comparative group Over 25% of bowel diaries incomplete Severity of symptoms varied widely in this small group Participants self selecting Unclear whether responses were linked to bowel changes or general health improvement

Terms: PMR: Progressive muscle relaxation; HADS: Hospital Anxiety & Depression Scale; HCAMQ: Holistic Complementary & Alternative Medicine Questionnaire; SAI: State Anxiety Inventory; STAI: State Trait Anxiety Inventory; CES–D: Centre for Epidemiological Studies Depression Scale; SCL-90: Symptom Checklist-90 Revised. MBSRQ-MS: Multidimensional Body-Self Relations Questionnaire – modified for multiple sclerosis; IFST-MS: Inventory of Functional Status-Multiple Sclerosis; C-GHQ-12/28: (Chinese) General Health Questionnaire; SF-36: Short Form Health Status; HAT: Hostile Automatic Thoughts Scale; BP: Blood Pressure; HR: Heart Rate; WHQ: Women's Health Questionnaire; MS: Multiple Sclerosis; PD: Parkinson's Disease; VAS: Visual Analogue Scale; PMS: Pre Menstrual Syndrome; FLI: Functional Living Index – Cancer Scale; PS: Performance Scale; PSS: Perceived Stress Scale; Image-SP: Illness image self profile; DQ: discharge questionnaire; C-STAI: Chinese State-Trait Anxiety Inventory. Qol-Colostomy: Quality of Life Index for Colostomy; WHOQoL: World Health Organisation Quality of Life Scale; AIMS2: Arthritis Impact Measures.

may have biased the responses. Similarly, Boyd et al. (2001) undertook a pilot study (n=6) of semi-structured interviews with six clients after six sessions of reflexology and identified the following themes: improvements related to the reflexology, sense of relaxation, interest in self-care, feeling cared for/time for self and reactions related to areas treated on the feet. The researcher, a mental health nurse, noted that many of the conversations were 'far more meaning-ful and detailed', precisely because talking was incidental to the intervention and acknowledged reliance on her nursing skills to create and maintain a safe and therapeutic relationship. However, whilst data from these types of study suggest that reflexology might be beneficial, these are retrospective accounts with little opportunity to evaluate other factors which may have influenced the reported outcome, a fact which does not provide conclusive evidence for the effectiveness of reflexology.

OBSERVATIONAL STUDIES

Case studies, which report individual observations, or large prospective cohort studies in which groups are observed over time, can provide valu-able data. For example, the individual reactions to reflexology of a group of patients with a specific symptom/condition may be collated. Both types of observational study have validity, but lack of a control group or an alternative treatment arm precludes evaluation of the specific effects of reflexology com-pared with other aspects of the treatment session, e.g. time and attention from a therapist (a non-specific effect). Such studies may provide useful data on the experience of having reflexology, and could inform future research ques-tions, but cannot be claimed as conclusive evidence of effectiveness, since the patient's condition may have resolved spontaneously (Ernst 2002: 13). In 1996, Vickers suggested that therapists only report successful studies and not fail-ures, although there are some reports of unresponsive cases and incidents when patients chose to discontinue treatment (Tiran 1996; Mackereth 1999).

LABORATORY EXPERIMENTS

This approach affords the researcher greater control over the variables that in 'real world' research may affect the results. For example, researchers can precisely control conditions such as room temperature, study duration and chemical mixes (Cook & Campbell 1997). In reflexology, White et al. (2000) conducted a study with two practitioners blinded to (unaware of) the medical diagnosis of 18 subjects, aiming to assess the ability of reflexologists to make a diagnosis by foot palpation only; no dialogue or history-taking was permit-ted. However, while the results showed that reflexology was not successful in identifying a diagnosis, this conclusion was based on a sample of only two reflexologists, yet it is estimated that there are more than 12 000 reflexologists in the UK (Mills & Budd 2000). It is possible that these *practitioners* were inef-fective in such controlled conditions, rather than the *therapy*, particularly as the controls placed on the study did not reflect normal reflexology practice, in which practitioners have longer to observe reactions and to gather data on the treatment responses. It is argued that reflexology practice is a 'package' with a number of factors influencing assessment, interventions and outcomes

Reflexology: expanding the evidence

experienced by patients and that, in trying to isolate specific components, the relationship between these factors may be lost to the researcher.

RANDOMISED CONTROLLED TRIALS

As with any form of research enquiry, the method adopted must be appropriate for the question to be answered, and not driven by the therapy under scrutiny or its philosophical foundations. If the research question aims to evaluate effectiveness, then a method is required which enables one to attribute *any* effect specifically to the intervention. The double-blind, randomised, controlled trial (RCT) is claimed to be the 'gold standard' in providing evidence of this type (Mercer et al. 1995). Most mainstream healthcare purchasers and providers believe that interventions must be subject to such scrutiny before being available in clinical practice.

RCTs are concerned with examining a causal relationship between intervention and outcome. Typically, participants are randomly allocated to one of two groups; one receives a placebo and the other the intervention being investigated, with the patient, his or her physician and the researcher being blinded to the allocation (Oldham 1994). The primary strength of the RCT is that it reduces bias through this random allocation of participants, which ensures that the groups being compared differ only by chance. However, the RCT has been subject to criticism, especially in respect of complementary medicine research (Vincent & Furnham 1997), although these criticisms can equally be levied at orthodox medical trials. Problems include feasibility of blinding, artificial standardisation of treatment, overstringent inclusion criteria resulting in non-representativeness of trial participants, ethical dilemmas associated with placebo treatments, participation affecting behaviour and therefore outcome, failure to take into account individual variations in responses to treatment and overemphasis on group effects.

It is argued that blinding of treatment is not possible for many CAM therapies, particularly those requiring manipulation or massage, including reflexology, since the patient is aware of being touched. Certainly, this presents a challenge, as an experienced reflexologist makes an autonomous decision about treatment which is appropriate to the individual. Standardising treatment may remove some of the elements integral to the therapeutic encounter, such as the client–therapist relationship. Therapeutic effectiveness should, therefore, be judged by an assessment of the whole encounter, and not restricted to the physical effects of the therapy alone. Further, evaluation of standardised treatment would be far removed from day-to-day practice; thus, results may have little clinical application.

Blinding participants to the treatment they receive aims to control for psychological components of the placebo effect, i.e. to ensure that treatment does not work only because participants expect it to (Carter 2003). However, practitioners would argue that reflexology is designed to benefit both body and mind. There is evidence to support the notion of an interactive relationship between the brain and immune system (e.g. Clow & Hucklebridge 2002). Thus, if participants were not aware of the treatment they received, the full potential for healing would not be harnessed. It is also possible that some patients may have a treatment preference and, if allocated to the control group, may feel that they had 'drawn the short straw', leading to disillusionment which could exaggerate the real benefit of a therapy (Cook & Campbell 1997). Therefore, it is important to provide an alternative treatment arm where these contextual elements exist for both interventions, for example all participants having the same treatment time and the attention of a therapist.

Researchers have attempted to include control groups in which the participants receive 'sham' (false) reflexology. These have included 'uneven tactile stimulation' on reflex points unrelated to the symptoms being investigated (Olesen & Flocco 1993); reflexology to a 'non-specific zone' (Lafeuente et al. 1990) and calf massage (Siev-Ner et al. 1997), although any touch techniques to the feet might have an influence on reflexology zones (Petersen et al. 1992).

The controlled trial by Williamson et al. (2002) of 76 women with menopausal symptoms randomised participants to two parallel arms; reflexology or non-specific foot massage. Both groups had similar attrition rates, and demonstrated improvements in mood, frequency of flushes and night sweats. However, blinding participants proved problematic, with 14 women reporting that they recognised whether they were receiving massage or reflexology, despite claiming no previous experience of reflexology at the start of the trial. This suggests that a control treatment of 'sham' reflexology is inappropriate in the study design. However, despite the criticisms levelled at RCTs, they remain the most accepted method for evidence of effectiveness of interventions. If reflexology is to be accepted by mainstream healthcare providers, further evidence from well-designed RCTs will need to be provided.

WHAT IS THE CURRENT STATE OF THE EVIDENCE FOR REFLEXOLOGY?

Poole (2001) previously reviewed evidence from controlled reflexology studies up to the year 2000, but it is encouraging that much more reflexology research has been published since then. Table 6.1 summarises key research evidence for reflexology from 2000–2009 and contains controlled studies, case reports and qualitative studies, as well as some studies of hand reflexology, some of which combined reflexology with foot massage. Interested readers are encouraged to pursue the original references for more detail.

The list is not exhaustive, but reflects the majority of reflexology studies since 2000. High-quality controlled studies remain limited and many studies cover a range of conditions and populations, making them difficult to summarise. Furthermore, it is apparent that many studies are methodologically flawed. Nevertheless, if we consider solely the controlled studies, several provide some evidence of effectiveness of reflexology in the context of cancer, pain and anxiety, although there are as many others which do not. An absence of evidence of effectiveness does not mean that the treatment is ineffective – it simply means there is no evidence to date to demonstrate that effectiveness. More, better-quality studies are needed if reflexology is to become more widely available within general healthcare settings. Clearly, reflexology is a complex intervention, provided by therapists with differing training and experience and accessed by patients with a range of health and well-being concerns.

Some additional recommendations for consideration by future researchers are shown below:

- Consider multicentred trials to recruit larger samples, if conditions are feasible and protocols can be adhered to.
- Consider measuring physiological and biological markers outside the treatment period and over the longer term, to investigate cumulative rather than transient effects.
- Consider incorporating qualitative approaches (e.g. interviews, focus groups, diaries) to provide more specific information on the views of individuals with complex and changeable health problems and their experience of reflexology (a complex intervention).
- Consider who provides the intervention (e.g. lay therapists compared to health professionals providing reflexology, partners/family members compared to trained reflexologists).

ETHICAL ISSUES

No discussion of research design and methods would be complete without mention of ethical issues. Archer (1999) argues that researchers need to consider moral and ethical concerns, given that both efficacy and – crucially – safety are key questions when making decisions about healthcare services. The concepts of beneficence and non-maleficence (see Ch. 4) are fundamental to ethical clinical practice and to clinical research activities.

Ethical guidelines for research focus on protecting participants' rights to ensure that individual autonomy is respected and they are treated fairly (Dresden et al. 2003); these are broadly similar across the health and social care sectors. However, the process of obtaining ethical approval can be different dependent upon the setting. In England, before commencing any research involving NHS staff, patients or locations, approval from a local Research Ethics Committee and a Research Governance Committee is necessary. If the research is related to an educational institution, (e.g. a student undertaking a research project), ethics approval from the university will also be required. The procedures can appear daunting to the novice researcher, but they are essential and are designed to protect both the researcher and the participants (see Further Resources).

Before submitting their research protocol for ethical approval, researchers must consider all the potential ethical issues in their project, beginning by questioning their motives for the research. Healthcare workers/researchers must consider the benefits for the wider community and recognise that, while the research may enhance their prestige and career advancement, its primary goal is to improve the welfare of the community (Weijer 1999). Research investigating effectiveness and/or safety would comply with this.

The main ethical issues are those of informed consent, patient privacy, confidentiality and the right to withdraw from the study. Participants have the right to know:

- who is conducting the research
- the purpose of the research
- how it is being funded
- what participation will involve
- any risks and benefits in taking part

- how any information they give will be treated
- that they have the right to withdraw from the study at any time without giving a reason
- what will happen to their data should they withdraw from the study.

They also have the right to expect:

- that any information they give will be treated in the strictest confidence,
- that data will be anonymised and stored responsibly
- that confidentiality will be maintained.

This information helps them to make an informed choice about whether or not to consent to participate. The written information should also contain sources of further information, impartial advice and the procedure for dealing with complaints. Once they have had the opportunity to ask questions and have decided that they would like to participate, they will be in a position to give informed consent. Ethically, the concept of 'informed consent' is a misnomer, since the patient cannot possibly be given complete information about all the possible outcomes. Complementary therapies such as reflexology are claimed to be individualised, which presents challenges to researchers when fully describing the benefits and risks. However, the treatment should be represented fairly and honestly, without bias and acknowledging any limitations in the current evidence, so that patients can make as informed a choice as possible.

CONCLUSION

Research is essential for the future development of the reflexology profession. Despite reflexology's long history, research in the discipline is still relatively young, although the increase in the number and calibre of recent studies is encouraging. However, there is still much work to be done in generating evidence for effectiveness in different populations and for different conditions. It is hoped that some practitioners will be encouraged to become involved in research, as it is only via the involvement of practitioners with the knowledge and expertise to design studies with appropriate methodology that reflexology can develop its professionalism and gain acceptance in the wider healthcare community.

REFERENCES

Archer, C., 1999. Research issues in complementary therapies. Complement. Ther. Nurs. Midwifery 5 (4), 108–114.

Boyd, D., Evans, C., Drennan, V., 2001. Using reflexology: a feasibility study. Ment. Health Nurs. 21 (6), 4–16.

Brown, C.A., Lido, C., 2008. Reflexology treatment for patients with lower limb amputations and phantom limb pain: an exploratory pilot study. Complement. Ther. Clin. Practice 14, 124–131.

Carter, B., 2003. Methodological issues and complementary therapies: researching intangibles? Complement. Ther. Nurs. Midwifery 9, 133–139.

Clow, A., Hucklebridge, F. (Eds.), 2002. Neurobiology of the immune system. Academic Press: an imprint of Elsevier Science, London.

Cook, T.D., Campbell, D.T., 1997. Quasi-experimentation and analysis for field settings. Houghton Mifflin, London.

Dresden, E., McElmurry, B.J., McCreary, L.L., 2003. Approaching ethical reasoning in nursing research through a communitarian perspective. J. Prof. Nurs. 19 (5), 295–304.

Ernst, E., 2002. Evidence-based massage therapy: a contradiction in terms? In: Rich, G.J. (Ed.), Massage therapy: the evidence for practice. Mosby, London.

Gambles, M., Crooke, M., Wilkinson, S., 2002. Evaluation of a hospice based reflexology service: a qualitative audit of patient perceptions. Eur. J. Oncol. Nurs. 6 (1), 37–44.

Grealish, L., Lomasny, A., Whiteman, B., 2000. Foot massage: a nursing intervention to modify the distressing symptoms of pain and nausea in patients hospitalised with cancer. Cancer Nursing 23 (3), 237–243.

Gunnarsdottir, J.T., Jonsdottir, H., 2007. Does the experimental design capture the effects of complementary therapy? A study using reflexology for patients undergoing coronary artery bypass graft surgery. J. Clin. Nurs. 16, 777–785.

Hodgson, H., 2000. Does reflexology impact on cancer patient's quality of life? Nurs. Stand. 14 (31), 33–38.

Hodgson, N.A., Andersen, S., 2008. The clinical efficacy of reflexology in nursing home residents with dementia. J. Altern. Complement. Med. 14 (3), 269–275.

House of Lords Select Committee on Science and Technology, 2000. 6th Report on Complementary & Alternative Medicine. HL. 118. HMSO, London.

Lafeuente, A., Noguera, M., Puy, C., Molins, A., Titus, F., Sans, F., 1990. Effekt der refllexzone behandlung am fuss bezuglich der prophylaktischen behandlung mit funarizin bei an cephalea-kopfscmerzen leidenden patienten. Erfahrungsheilkunde 39, 713–715.

Mackereth, P.A., 1999. An introduction to catharsis and the healing crisis in reflexology. Complement. Ther. Nurs. Midwifery 5 (3), 67–74.

Mackereth, P.A., Booth, K., Hillier, V.F., Caress, A.-L., 2009a. Reflexology and progressive muscle relaxation training for people with multiple sclerosis: A cross trial. Complement. Ther. Clin. Pract. 15, 14–21.

Mackereth, P.A., Booth, K., Hillier, V.F., Caress, A.-L., 2009b. What do people talk about during reflexology? Analysis of worries and concerns expressed during sessions for patients with multiple sclerosis. Complement. Ther. Clin. Pract. 15, 85–90.

McNeill, J.A., Alderdice, F.A., McMurray, F., 2006. A retrospective cohort study exploring the relationship between antenatal reflexology and intranatal outcomes. Complement. Ther. Clin. Pract. 12, 119–125.

McVicar, A.J., Greenwood, C.R., Fewell, F., D'Arcy, V., Chandrasekharan, S., Aldridge, L.C., 2007. Evaluation of anxiety, salivary cortisol and melatonin secretion following reflexology treatment: a pilot study in healthy individuals. Complement. Ther. Clin. Pract. 13, 137–145.

Mercer, G., Long, A.F., Smith, I.J., 1995. Researching and evaluating complementary therapies: the state of the debate. Nuffield Institute for Health, University of Leeds, Leeds, UK.

Mills, S., Budd, S., 2000. Professional organisation of complementary and alternative medicine in the United Kingdom. Centre for the Complementary Health Studies, University of Exeter, Exeter, UK.

Mollart, L., 2003. Single-blind trial addressing the differential effects of two reflexology techniques versus rest, on ankle and foot oedema in late pregnancy. Complement. Ther. Nurs. Midwifery 9, 203–208.

Oldham, J., 1994. Experimental and quasi-experimental research designs. Nurse Res. 1 (4), 26–36.

Olesen, T., Flocco, W., 1993. Randomized controlled study of pre-menstrual symptoms treated with ear, hand and foot reflexology. Obstet. Gynecol. 82 (6), 906–911.

Peterson, L.N., Faurschou, P., Olsen, O.T., Svendsen, U.G., 1992. Foot zone therapy and bronchial asthma: a controlled clinical trial. Ugeskr. Laeger 154 (30), 2065–2068.

Poole, H., 2001. Researching reflexology. In: Mackereth, P., Tiran, D. (Eds.), Clinical reflexology: a guide for health professionals. Churchill Livingstone, London.

Poole, H., Glenn, S., Murphy, P., 2007. A randomised controlled study of reflexology for the management of chronic low back pain. Eur. J. Pain 11, 878–887.

Quattrin, R., Zanini, A., Buchini, S., Turello, D., Annunziata, M.A., Vidotti Colombatti, A., et al., 2006. Use of reflexology foot massage to reduce anxiety in hospitalized cancer patients in chemotherapy treatment: methodology and outcomes. J. Nurs. Manag. 14, 96–105.

Quinn, F., Hughes, C.M., Baxter, G.D., 2008. Reflexology in the management of low back pain: a pilot randomised controlled trial. Complement. Ther. Med. 16, 3–8.

Sackett, D.L., Rosenberg, W.M.C., Gray, J.A.M., Hayne, R.B., Richardson, W.S., 1996. Evidence based medicine: what it is and what it isn't. BMJ 312, 196–203.

Siev-Ner, I., Gamus, D., Lerner-Geva, L., Azaria, M., Sha'ked, D., Zaidel, S., 1997. Reflexology treatment relieves symptoms of multiple sclerosis: a randomized controlled study. Focus Alternat. Complement. Ther. 2, 196.

Smith, G., 2002. A randomised controlled clinical trial of reflexology in breast cancer patients, to reduce fatigue resulting from radiotherapy to the breast and chest wall. PhD thesis, University of Liverpool, Liverpool (unpublished).

Stephenson, N.L.N., Weinrich, S.P., 2000. The effects of foot reflexology on anxiety and pain in patients with breast and lung cancer. Oncol. Nurs. Forum 27 (1), 67–72.

Stephenson, N., Dalton, J.A., Carlson, J., 2003. The effect of foot reflexology on pain in patients with metastatic cancer. Appl. Nurs. Res. 16 (4), 284–286 35, 37–47.

Stephenson, N.L.N., Swanson, M., Dalton, J., Keefe, E.F., Engelke, M., 2007. Partner-delivered reflexology: effects on cancer pain and anxiety. Oncol. Nurs. Forum 34 (1), 127–132.

Tiran, D., 1996. The use of complementary therapies in midwifery practice: a focus on reflexology. Complement. Ther. Nurs. Midwifery 2 (2), 32–37.

Tovey, P., 2002. A single-blind trial of reflexology for irritable bowel syndrome. Br. J. Gen. Pract. 52 (474), 19–23.

Vickers, A., 1996. Massage and aromatherapy: a guide for health professionals. Chapman & Hall, London.

Vincent, C., Furnham, A., 1997. Complementary medicine: a research perspective. John Wiley & Sons, Chicester, UK.

Weijer, C., 1999. Selecting subjects for participation in clinical research: one sphere of justice. J. Med. Ethics 25, 31–36.

White, A.R., Williamson, J., Hart, A., Ernst, E., 2000. A blinded investigation into the accuracy of reflexology charts. Complement. Ther. Med. 8, 166–172.

Wilkinson, I.S., Prigmore, S., Rayner, C.F., 2006. A randomised-controlled trial examining the effects of reflexology on patients with chronic obstructive pulmonary disease (COPD). Complement. Ther. Clin. Practice 12, 141–147.

Williamson, J., White, A., Hart, A., Ernst, E., 2002. Randomized controlled trial of reflexology for menopausal symptoms. BJOG 109, 1050–1055.

Woodward, S., Norton, C. Barriball, K., 2009. (in press). A pilot study of the effectiveness of reflexology in treating idiopathic constipation in women. Complement. Ther. Clin. Pract. (accessed 9 Sept 2009).

Wyatt, G., Sikorskii, A., Siddiqi, A., Given, C.W., 2007. Feasibility of a reflexology and guided imagery intervention during chemotherapy: results of a quasi-experimental study. Oncol. Nurs. Forum 34 (3), 635–642.

Reflexology: expanding the evidence

FURTHER READING

Hymel, G., 2006. Research methods for massage and holistic therapies. Churchill Livingstone, London.

Polgar, S., Thomas, S.A., 2008. Introduction to research in the health sciences. Churchill Livingstone, London.

USEFUL RESOURCES

The Research Council for Complementary Medicine website has information on research design, courses and funding opportunities, http://www.rccm.org.uk/default.aspx?m=0.

The National Center for Complementary and Alternative Medicine an American website with information on many therapies and pages on research design and funding, http://nccam.nih.gov/.

NHS Ethics: http://www.nres.npsa.nhs.uk/ contains guidance on how to apply and links to further information on ethics in health.

NHS Research Governance and Ethics, http://www.dh.gov.uk/en/Researchanddevelopment/A-Z/Researchgovernance/index.htm.

Revisiting the 'rules' of reflexology

7

Denise Tiran

ABSTRACT

Reflexology has become more professionalised, more evidence-based and more integrated into some specialisms within mainstream healthcare, and some of the traditional ideas, which were a feature of reflexology practice for so long, have now been largely rejected, although this is by no means universal. This chapter explores some of the 'rules' and traditions of reflexology and challenges their validity in contemporary reflexology clinical practice, especially when reflexology is incorporated into mainstream healthcare.

KEY WORDS

Styles of reflexology, diagnosis, prescription, stimulation, reflexology techniques, reflexology charts.

INTRODUCTION

When one looks at its status within twenty-first-century mainstream health-care, reflexology is still an evolving profession, despite the work of various respected authorities who have worked tirelessly to promote its benefits and

81

DOI: 10.1016/B978-0-7020-3167-0.00007-X

to demonstrate that, by working in an integrated manner in conjunction with conventional healthcare professionals, the potential risks can be minimised. When complementary therapies are presented with clear expectations of outcomes, possible benefits and, most importantly, their limitations, they are usually welcomed into conventional healthcare. For example, most hospices and some NHS cancer hospitals in the UK employ complementary therapists as part of the multidisciplinary team, and cancer support centres offering complementary therapies are recognised as an integral part of community palliative care in many areas. Reflexology can be used to relieve pain, reduce symptoms associated with medical treatments and ease stress and the emotional aspects of life-limiting illness (Kohara et al. 2004; Williams et al. 2009). Similarly, reflexology and other complementary therapies are increasingly part of mainstream maternity care, particularly in view of the rising Caesarean section rates, and have been used to facilitate normal birth, relieve physiological symptoms of pregnancy and aid adaptation to parenthood (Tiran 2009). Another clinical field in which complementary therapies such as reflexology have become popular is that of learning disability care, calming and relaxing clients, improving mobility and enhancing quality of life (Gale & Hegarty 2000).

However, although research evidence remains limited (see Ch. 6), reflexologists do their profession no favours by making exaggerated claims based on anecdotal evidence, and the medical profession sometimes finds it difficult to accept complementary therapies which are accompanied by unscientific and unlikely explanations and unevaluated enthusiasms. Research, audit and collation of clinical evidence can contribute to the acquisition of new information about the benefits and potential side effects associated with reflexology, especially in relation to specific clinical groups. It could be argued that it is no longer entirely appropriate to consider reflexology solely as a relaxation modality, but to acknowledge that it is an extremely powerful and valuable tool in its own right, which can be added to other tools used in both conventional medicine and complementary healthcare.

'RULES' IN REFLEXOLOGY PRACTICE

Various 'rules' have traditionally been included in reflexology training and were intended as a means of protecting both clients and therapists. Some *guidelines* for practice are included at pre-registration level but, following qualification as a reflexologist, further training and experience enable the boundaries of safe practice to be stretched. For example, therapists in training are often discouraged from treating women in the first trimester of pregnancy, yet there are many midwives and some therapists who now treat women for problems which occur in very early pregnancy (see Ch. 9). Other 'rules' are based on differences in legal definitions and the current regulatory status of reflexologists in relation to conventional healthcare professionals (see Ch. 4). Greater integration of complementary therapies into orthodox healthcare has resulted in in-depth explorations of basic and post-basic training, regulation, insurance and other issues, which are gradually producing highly competent and knowledgeable practitioners, able to take their place with credibility and professionalism in the wider healthcare arena (see Ch. 3). Debate continues surrounding the issues of standardisation within the reflexology profession, not least the need to work together to clarify traditional beliefs about the therapy, to consider uniformity of reflexology charts and to challenge variations in practice and theoretical principles which underpin practice. Let us, then, explore further some of these 'rules' that have previously placed somewhat unnecessary restrictions on practice but which are now being seen less as mandatory parameters for practice and more as guidelines which can be questioned and adapted on condition that the practitioner is able to justify his or her actions.

STANDARDISATION

STYLES OF REFLEXOLOGY AND VARIATIONS IN CHARTS

One of the difficulties for the generic profession of reflexology is that there are so many styles of practice, from 'salon' reflexology for general relaxation, to clinical reflex zone therapy for the treatment of specific conditions, from the very scientific focus of new styles such as Adapted Reflextherapy (see Ch. 11) to methods with a more traditional and esoteric background such as Five Element reflexology. If reflexology was purely an artistic discipline it would be acceptable to have many different styles, as we see in painting, with modernist, impressionist, fauvist and so on. However, reflexology is also a scientific discipline requiring sound knowledge accumulated through systematic study and organised by general principles. It is, perhaps, the wide variations in styles and theories which cause many conventional healthcare professionals – and some reflexologists – to challenge the validity of reflexology practice in academic and scientific terms. Whilst it is interesting to have different schools of thought which facilitate rich academic debate aimed at progressing professional practice, the existence of so many differing styles makes it difficult to standardise the profession without compromising some authorities. However, ongoing debate contributes to the development of a more cohesive profession, and increasingly the fundamental principles which are common to most styles of reflexology are debated, tested, researched, practiced and evaluated.

General reflexology is primarily a relaxation therapy which aims to restore homeostasis. Many schools teach the Ingham method™ which is based on the original work of Eunice Ingham and her nephew, Dwight Byers, using techniques which were formerly termed 'compression massage of the feet'. Vertical reflexology, adapted from the Ingham method™, uses reflex points on the dorsal surfaces of the hands and feet to treat clients whilst in a temporary weight-bearing position which is thought to facilitate stimulation of deeper reflex points, enabling therapeutic effects in a shorter period of time. Precision reflexology (see Ch. 14) builds on general reflexology, using a process known as 'linking' in which two or three reflexology points are held simultaneously to enhance its overall impact and to enable treatment of specific conditions. In synergistic reflexology the hand and foot are worked simultaneously and several points are worked together, as in precision reflexology. These forms of reflexology have a similar theoretical basis and use largely the same charts, albeit with minor adaptations to suit the individual style.

Reflex zone therapy (RZT) is a specific clinical modality and can be administered in what might be accused of as being reductionist, rather than holistic, with short focused treatments according to the precise health needs of the individual. Whilst it has the same basic principles embedded within its theoretical background, reflex zone therapy has a more Western conventional scientific approach than some other forms of reflexology. The Metamorphic technique, an off-shoot of RZT, focuses primarily on the foot zones corresponding to the spine, thought to reflect a time period related to the nine months of intrauterine life; treatment aims to correct imbalances thought to be caused by activities occurring both before and immediately after birth. In a similar manner, spinal reflexology acknowledges the neurological link between the spinal vertebrae and specific nerves, organs, muscles, etc., but in this method the therapist uses the hands and thumbs on the client's back to identify which vertebrae are out of balance so that both the affected organ(s) and the nerves that serve the organ are treated.

Whilst the philosophy and mechanism of action are considered to be similar in many styles of general reflexology, some schools teach a method which is more closely linked to the meridians of Chinese medicine, based on the notion of energy lines (meridians) linking one part of the body to another. This type of reflexology requires an understanding of Eastern philosophies and knowledge of the meridians as used in acupuncture. It includes Chi reflexology, a relative newcomer, which was developed by Moss Arnold, and the ancient Five Element reflexology incorporating yin–yang balance and the elements of fire, water, metal, wood and earth. A Japanese form, Zoku shin do, thought to be over 5000 years old, also focuses on yin–yang harmony and balance. Vacuflex reflexology™, a modern system of treatment, combines meridian rebalancing and reflex point stimulation via suction boots on the feet, and suction cups on other parts of the body attached to a suction pump.

Some forms of reflexology use techniques in which the pressure applied to the foot is adapted to suit the theory underpinning the particular school of thought. The Advanced Reflexology Technique (ART™) devised by Tony Porter focuses on the precise *texture* of reflex points, with pressure being deeper than in many other styles of reflexology, although that used in RZT is considerably firmer than in generic reflexology. An even firmer pressure is used in the Taiwanese Rwo Shur, in which treatment is applied using not only the hands but also wooden or plastic bars and a special cream to reduce friction. Conversely, in Morrell reflex touch, an extremely light touch is used to activate both neurological and energy pathways, and the more contemporary Gentle Touch Reflexology™ is based on a belief, similar to that in homeopathy, that the more gentle (or 'dilute') the application, the more powerful it becomes. Other variations relate to whether or not creams, lotions or implements are used in the treatment: ART™ involves the application of special cream to enable the practitioner's hands to pass over the client's feet without friction, whereas in reflex zone therapy, creams, lotions or talcum powder are avoided, as it is felt that they may mask signs which can be clinically significant, e.g. the odour of the feet or the amount of perspiration on them.

Several styles combine aspects of other therapies, for example SMART Ayurvedic Reflexology is a blend of the reflex maps of foot reflexology and a special foot massage routine used in Indian Ayurvedic medicine, using oils selected according to the individual's energy balance and incorporating meridian work. Other styles are emerging in which the reflexology maps of the feet are used as a medium through which to apply different therapeutic interventions, as in Foot-applied Bowen therapy (see Ch. 14). Coordinative Reflexology, an Israeli therapy devised in the 1980s, incorporates a series of flowing techniques similar to dance and may involve treatment being given by one or two practitioners. Integrative reflexology encompasses the zones and reflex points of traditional reflexology, as well as the inter-relationships linked by the body's meridians and proprioceptors, together with structural alignment techniques based on the manual therapy of rolfing. Structural reflex zone therapy (see Ch. 14; Tiran 2009) is theoretically based both on the principles of RZT and those of osteopathy, in which the body is assessed in terms of musculoskeletal misalignment, and the reflex zones on the feet are used as a medium through which to realign any significant deviations. Adapted reflextherapy (see Ch. 11) is also based on the RZT model, but has a specific application to physiotherapy practice, although it can be applied to other clinical specialisms if appropriate.

These many styles each differ slightly from each other, which can be challenging to practitioners and confusing to sceptics who seek to denigrate reflexology and to reject the notion of a cohesive profession of reflexology. At an academic level the variations between styles can be exciting and fascinating, but one could argue that, until we have a greater degree of uniformity within reflexology, we are in danger of never being able to standardise practice, theory or research, since different practitioners may approach their work from different perspectives from that of their colleagues. The charts used by different schools have minor or – in some cases – major variations, with reflex points varying considerably, which has to be a fundamental issue needing resolution before we can develop further. Perhaps what we can see evolving in contemporary practice is a range of different therapies which are *based on* reflexology, but which are, in fact, individual therapies in their own right.

DIAGNOSIS AND PRESCRIPTION

The issue of whether or not complementary practitioners should 'diagnose' has hitherto fuelled much debate, not just amongst reflexologists. The word 'diagnosis' originates from the Greek *dia* meaning 'through' and *gnosis* meaning 'knowledge' and an 'investigation or analysis of the *cause* or *nature of* a condition' (Merriam Webster Medical Dictionary 2009), 'the discovery and identification of diseases from the examination of symptoms' (Collins Online Dictionary 2006), or, more recently, 'the act or process of identifying or determining the nature and cause of a disease or injury through evaluation of a patient history, examination and review of laboratory data' (American Heritage Dictionary of English Language Online 2009).

In relation to complementary therapies in general and to reflexology in particular, the UK situation regarding diagnosis by therapists is compounded by the European Community's reliance on Napoleonic law in which the term 'diagnosis' refers to a process undertaken only by qualified medical practitioners. However, 'analysis of the cause or nature of a condition' does not necessarily imply attaching a specific title or label to a set of signs and symptoms, but can apply in general terms and to that part of the process which leads to a conclusion. In medical practice, it is not always possible for a single individual or discipline to reach a conclusion in isolation, and a team approach may be needed to document the data and combine their ideas in order to reach a diagnosis. There are, in addition, different categories of diagnosis, including 'clinical diagnosis' based on signs, symptoms and laboratory tests, and 'differential diagnosis' whose signs and/or symptoms are shared by various other conditions. A contemporary list expanded to include allopathic diagnosis, complementary diagnosis and reflexology diagnosis would enhance the diagnostic potential for clients by drawing on the individualised skills of a multidisciplinary team (see Case Study 7.1).

CASE STUDY 7.1

A general practitioner (GP) referred a young mother for reflexology for migraine and depression. Initial assessment identified a constant 'fuzzy' head, 'gritty' eyes and perpetual tiredness to add to her depression, and inspection of the feet revealed a candidial infection of the toenail. During the next four treatments the reflex area for the thyroid gland became progressively more tender and palpable. The reflexologist sent a letter to the GP suggesting blood tests for thyroid dysfunction. However, soon afterwards, further research during a programme of personal study caused the practitioner to appreciate that all the mother's symptoms, including the toenail infection, were signs of underactive parathyroid glands (indistinguishably in the same reflex area as the thyroid) and he contacted the GP again to suggest tests for parathyroid gland function, with subsequent positive results. Vitamin D treatment was commenced along with continued reflexology and the client quickly recovered and progressed. This demonstrates the integrated diagnostic power of reflexology and conventional medicine and the importance of continuing professional development.

There is no doubt that reflexology, in the hands of an experienced practitioner, can contribute to the overall conclusions which need to be drawn before attempting to treat individual clients, and some preliminary work has been undertaken on the use of reflexology to aid diagnosis (White et al. 2000; Tiran & Chummun 2005). It is, of course, the very potential of reflexology to locate specific reflex zones on the feet (or hands), directly related to distal areas of the body that may be pathologically affected, that makes reflexology a useful diagnostic aid in clinical practice. It is, however, essential that the reflexologist has sufficient knowledge to interpret correctly the signs from the feet and the symptoms reported by the client to assist in making a diagnosis from which a decision can be made regarding appropriate treatment to be undertaken. The knowledge required is both complementary and conventional – indeed, it is this which sets *clinical reflexology* aside from typical 'salon reflexology'.

What makes 'diagnosis' difficult for newly qualified or inexperienced therapists is often a lack of full understanding of the implications of changes in a specific reflex zone, especially when the changes represent physiological or pathological changes. Furthermore, practitioners need to have an in-depth knowledge of anatomy, physiology and relevant pathology to avoid misinterpreting visual or palpatory nuances in the feet. This understanding may seem less imperative when a therapist agrees to treat a referral from a doctor who has already decided that the patient's conditions warrants reflexology treatment. However, it is an unfortunate fact that many doctors do not have adequate awareness or willingness to be able to refer for reflexology with authority, highlighting the need for reflexologists to be trained to make these decisions independently. This has become a much more urgent requirement of late, since the litigation-conscious society in which we live is keen to apportion blame for errors brought to court by patients or clients who are dissatisfied with their care.

It must be stressed that there is *no* claim that reflexology techniques alone can furnish a diagnosis, at least not in allopathic terms. A study by Raz et al. (2003) found that reflexology can only be considered a reliable method of diagnosis in those systems with organs in an exact location. In other words, it may be possible to be alerted to changes in a specific organ such as the stomach, but not to identify a systemic condition such as hypertension. Furthermore, the practitioner would need to be able to differentiate between changes which are physiological (in this case, digestion), those which may occur as a result of the reflexology treatment (increased peristalsis) and those which may be impending or actual pathological problems (for example, irritable bowel syndrome).

On the subject of diagnosis, the core curriculum for reflexology (O'Hara 2006) affirms that students should not presume to furnish an allopathic label to the client's condition, even if their observation and treatment of the feet, in conjunction with the client's history, suggests a particular condition. However, in order to embark on a course of therapeutic action, the practitioner must decide what he or she is going to do during the treatment session. This is, in essence, a prescription, which cannot be made without having first formed an idea of the client's condition (i.e. coming to a decision about a possible diagnosis) by whatever means. A 'prescription' is generally considered to be a written instruction from a doctor to a pharmacist for preparing and dispensing a drug. However, clinical reflexologists are qualified to 'prescribe' reflexology as a result of an assessment and to decide upon further treatments based on an evaluation of the client's condition so far, although it is essential that they acknowledge their professional boundaries. The core curriculum (O'Hara 2006) makes it clear that the only thing reflexologists are qualified to prescribe is reflexology, in that they prescribe a treatment after the initial consultation.

COMBINING THERAPIES

There is much debate regarding the issue of multiskilled professionals but short introductory sessions on other therapies such as nutrition, which may be included in basic training courses, do not equip a reflexologist to work also as a nutritional therapist. On the other hand, if, because of such awareness of nutrition, a serious deficiency in a client's diet becomes evident during treatment, it would be irresponsible to ignore this. If the practitioner is additionally qualified to provide nutritional or other advice, perhaps a separate appointment could be offered, as a change of 'hat' helps the client to identify the change of role. To monitor reflexology effectiveness without complication, some reflexologists choose to refer such clients to another nutritional therapist.

Conversely, the combination of therapies can work synergistically for the client's well-being and should not be discounted. In addition, we must not overlook the client's prerogative to choose which therapy they receive, or the opportunity to document evidence-based practice and research. There must be acknowledgement that practitioners from other disciplines need to measure the effectiveness of their treatments, but as professional reflexologists, we need to be informed of the therapies that cannot be combined and be able to give a reasonable explanation as to why treatment combining is not always recommended. O'Hara (2008) challenged the views of some classical homeopaths and acupuncturists who actively discourage clients from combining therapies as this may complicate the clinical picture, particularly in respect of any claimed healing crisis (see Ch. 2) or side-effects. In general, reflexologists are taught that they should not combine different therapies. However, nurses and midwives who are appropriately trained in complementary therapies frequently combine various therapies, for example reflexology with aromatherapy and acupressure, and/or in conjunction with conventional medical treatment, as in maternity care (see Ch. 9) or treatment of those with addictions (see Ch. 13). Furthermore, developments within reflexology have elicited new treatment modalities in which the basic therapy is adapted and used in combination with aspects of other therapies, which are demonstrating marked benefits and effectiveness (see Ch. 14). The potential risks of interactions, side effects and the 'healing crisis' which occurs with reflexology and other therapies need to be taken into account, but this synergistic process can often be extremely beneficial and effective, although it may be good practice to advocate the principle of 'wearing one hat at a time' unless the practitioner is exceptionally experienced.

TREATING SPECIFIC CONDITIONS

When clients present with a specific condition, such as pain, neither complementary nor conventional practitioners can guarantee a cure. The terms 'treat' and 'cure' are often confused and practitioners should neither guarantee a resolution of the client's problems nor go to the opposite extreme and imply that reflexology treatment will be ineffective. The contemporary issue for those who persist in the view that they should not treat specific illnesses is the problem of participating in research studies designed with very specific parameters (see Ch. 6). Research projects such as 'the effect of reflexology on people with multiple sclerosis' (Siev-Ner et al. 2003) or 'a randomised controlled trial of premenstrual syndrome treated with reflexology' (Oleson & Flocco 1993) would not be possible if the reflexology strategy was generalised and unrelated to the specific condition. Reflexologists may indeed treat clients who happen to be suffering from specific conditions, but treatment should be within a holistic context where the client's own healing potential may be triggered by the treatment, thereby leading to alleviation in symptoms.

However, those who practice reflex zone therapy (RZT), according to the Marquardt style, would argue that their modality is consciously intended to treat people with specific conditions, particularly as, until relatively recently, entry to the profession of RZT was open only to conventional healthcare professionals and to osteopaths and chiropractors (professions which are now statutorily regulated and classified as 'supplementary to medicine', as opposed to 'complementary'). Practitioners of RZT differentiate between their therapy and generic reflexology by focusing on the fact that, as they are conventional healthcare professionals, usually working within mainstream healthcare settings, their clients present with health problems for which it is thought RZT may help. Textbooks on RZT give suggestions for treatment of specific conditions (Lett 2000; Marquardt 2000; Tiran 2009) although it is always emphasised that the practitioner is treating the *person* and not the *condition*, and that a formulaic approach to therapy is neither appropriate nor desirable. An example of this differentiation might be the focus on stress and stress-related conditions, which form a large part of generic reflexology practice. Of course, when treating a client with reflexology, we know that it can be calming and relaxing and this will facilitate a reduction in stress hormones (McVicar et al. 2007) which may indirectly impact on a pathological condition, such as hypertension, or on conditions in which high cortisol levels adversely affect health (see Ch. 1).

The treatment of specific conditions, however, requires a thorough working knowledge of physiology and pathology, which may not be well refined in reflexologists at the point of qualification and will only be deepened in those who choose to specialise in a particular clinical field. For example, practitioners who work in cancer care will have a level of knowledge about different types of tumours, and about the conventional treatment required; further, they will develop knowledge of how reflexology impacts on both the patient's condition and on the treatment (e.g. interactions). It is, however, illegal to claim or guarantee to 'cure' cancer; practitioners working in cancer care provide supportive treatment of the person and their symptoms, rather than treatment aimed at 'resolving' the cause, i.e. the condition. Similarly it is illegal for anyone other than a midwife or doctor, or one in training under supervision, to take sole responsibility for a mother during pregnancy and childbirth; thus, reflexologists who treat pregnant women are providing treatment which is *complementary* to that offered by midwives and doctors, not *alternative*.

STANDARDISING TERMINOLOGY

One of the ways in which a profession is defined is the use of terminology specific to its practice, but until reflexologists employ the same language there remains the potential for communication breakdown and misunderstanding. Similarly, although individuals will develop variations in practice, techniques need to conform to professionally accepted norms, so that one practitioner's appreciation of terms such as 'stimulation', commonly used in reflexology, is the same as another's.

One factor influencing many of the decisions to label a situation as a contraindication may stem from an unbalanced view of how reflexology works and an overzealous use of the verb 'to stimulate'. Reflex points of nerve endings at the point of contact are apparently 'stimulated' by reflexology; in other words, a therapeutic response is achieved from a particular action. Perhaps this should more correctly be referred to as 'normalisation', the promotion of homeostasis or homeodynamics. Greater understanding of this process should assist the practitioner in identifying pertinent contraindications.

It is often postulated that 'stimulation' of a particular reflex point for which the condition of the relevant organ is normal should not cause hyperactivity in the organ. For example, manipulation of the thyroid gland reflex point may facilitate thyroxin release in the case of an underactive gland, but inadvertently vigorous use of the same technique should not cause hyperthyroid activity, although this principle has been disputed in contemporary clinical practice related to maternity care (Tiran 2009). Indeed, overemphasising the notion of 'stimulation' can be misleading, resulting in unfortunate decisions in clinical practice based, perhaps, on a fear of exacerbating the client's condition. An example of this would be the decision not to treat people with cancer because of the fear of stimulating circulation and spreading the disease, yet there are many examples of reflexology being used safely and effectively for people suffering from the effects of the disease or the treatments.

However, there remains disparity amongst practitioners, with those who practice RZT vehemently challenging this concept (Lett 2000; Marquardt 2000; Tiran 2009). In RZT, *stimulation* is a specific technique designed to *increase* a physiological process, for example intestinal transit in the case of constipation, or pituitary output to initiate labour contractions. This second example is significant, because generic reflexologists are taught to apply a light circular motion over the pituitary reflex zone as part of a standard treatment, yet in the theory of RZT this would constitute stimulation, which may – as has been shown in clinical midwifery practice – exacerbate pituitary function. At the very least, this could result in early onset of a menstrual period in a female client, or, if the woman is pregnant, may cause premature labour. Conversely, the RZT technique of *sedation* aims to *decrease* a process, notably pain, but also overactivity of organs. Other techniques, some of which are shared with generic reflexology, include simple massage, draining, holding and sweeping. Structural RZT (see Ch. 14) adds manipulation as a specific technique, particularly applied to the reflex zones for the musculoskeletal system. In addition, RZT, structural RZT and adapted reflextherapy (see Ch. 11) highlight the specific therapeutic action of *doing nothing*.

Many students – and some teachers – appear to accept unquestioningly the 'rules' they are given, even when no justification for a particular practice can be offered. Students and qualified practitioners should not be afraid to question and challenge; indeed, thought-provoking discussions as part of continuing professional development courses can sometimes lead to changes in ideas and, ultimately, in clinical practice. Reflexology is not an exact science and there is much that is still not fully understood, including the mechanism of action (see Chs 1 and 2). Until we know more about the ways in which reflexology works it is almost impossible to standardise the charts used and to justify the treatment routines.

There are many variations between charts (or maps) used in reflexology which has been discussed elsewhere (see O'Hara 2002; Tiran 2009). This inconsistency between charts and the location of reflex zones/points illustrates the need for clinical reflexologists continually to challenge the rigour of their basic training and to recognise the importance of continuing professional development and of clinical research. Before reflexology diagnoses can be consistent, the charts mapping the reflex points must be standardised. Dissent continues amongst reflexology authorities over the precise location of a number of reflex zones, with opinions usually based on personal practice and experience, although it must also be said that, on occasions, teaching has merely followed traditional charts without question. Debate about these variations is essential to improving and standardising practice and to making reflexology a more credible profession in the eyes of those external to it.

There remains contention between authorities regarding the precise location of reflex zones for various organs, notably the 'solar' or coeliac plexus zone, which, according to zone theory, should be located in zone 1 where the two feet come together (Fig. 7.1), but it has traditionally been located in zone 3 of the plantar surface of each foot. In another example, a condition affecting the pituitary gland cannot be reliably suggested if the reflex zone for the pituitary gland differs from one practitioner's chart to another. The traditional siting for the pituitary gland zone is in the centre of the plantar hallux.

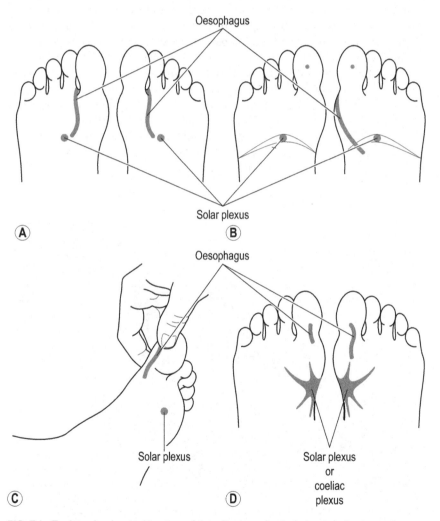

FIG. 7.1 Traditional and revised locations of the reflex zones for the 'solar plexus' and oesophagus according to (A) Dougans (1996), (B) Norman (1995), (C) Stormer (1992), (D) Lett (2000).

This also is not consistent with the zone arrangement, for the pituitary gland is anatomically in the centre of the head, so the pituitary reflex point should be in zone 1 of the foot, in common with the coeliac plexus. Reflexologists from most schools of thought have hitherto agreed that the pituitary reflex is at the 'peak' of the big toe 'where the whorl of the toe print converges into a central point', which, although differing from one client's toe shape to another, is usually in the centre of each big toe (Fig. 7.2). However, the majority of experts, teachers and practitioners have scant need to identify the precise location of the pituitary gland zone except when a pituitary condition may be manifest, and could easily make assumptions about their findings. On the other hand, midwives and those treating women during pregnancy and labour have a specific need to locate the relevant reflex zone correctly – either to avoid 'overstimulating' it during pregnancy (which, far from 'normalising' pituitary function may actually trigger abnormal hormonal production resulting in pregnancy complications), or to 'stimulate' the point in order to expedite contractions and the birth of the baby (Lett 2000; Marquardt 2000; Tiran 2009). Furthermore, correct positioning of the pituitary gland zone in non-pregnant women can facilitate accurate diagnosis of the stages of the menstrual cycle (Tiran & Chummun 2005). In direct contradiction to the testimony of other notable reflexology authorities, and to the traditional teachings of any other school, including RZT, Tiran (2009) places the pituitary gland reflex zone on the *outer edge* of the plantar surface of toe 1 on each foot. This seems entirely illogical, but is based on 25 years of experience of specifically treating pregnant women and is attributed to the possibility of 'working zones' from which the most appropriate clinical effects are achieved. This concept deserves further exploration when more evidence is available.

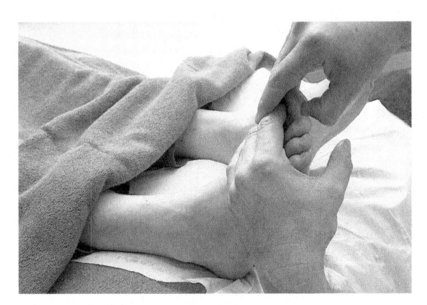

FIG. 7.2 Practitioner working the traditional reflex zone for the pituitary gland – see *Tiran Reflexology for Pregnancy and Childbirth* for debate on a possible new location. Photo courtesy of Katie Spruce BA (Hons), medical photographer, Christie Hospital NHS Trust, with permission.

The phenomenon of physical manifestations in the reflex zones of the feet also warrants some debate. An example is the often-quoted notion that a full bladder results in distension of the corresponding reflex points on the feet, although most tutors and practitioners would dispute this. On the other hand, many practitioners have become aware of changes in organs as a result of what they feel on palpation. It is generally accepted that 'deposits' or 'congestion' can be detected in reflex zones and they may provide us with some valuable information to assist in the treatment process. Conversely, focusing on using these 'deposits' to aid diagnosis could, in some instances, be very counterproductive, by changing the dynamics of a therapeutic partnership to one of paternalist didactic information-giving (see Ch. 5). This emphasises the intuitive element of reflexology and the need for a two-way communication between the practitioner and the client. The skill is in interpreting what is felt, and in understanding whether it represents changes in the actual reflex zone or whether it is simply the textural nature of the tissue. Perhaps the most reliable assessment of reflex zones is the sensitivity experienced by the client, who can then be involved in making the connection between the reflex zone and the corresponding body part, although Lett (2000) suggests that when the client has no sensation in a reflex zone this can be altogether more clinically significant, possibly indicating an as yet undiagnosed pathological problem. We do not know the exact nature of the 'grittiness' so often felt by practitioners, although many theories have been postulated. We do not know the extent to which this 'grittiness' is significant in clinical practice or whether it is simply a manifestation of changes which may, or may not, be pathological. For example, it is common to palpate an area of 'grittiness' around the reflex zones for the shoulders, which many therapists attribute to muscular tension in the shoulders, but which is considered to be relatively normal. However, palpating a similar deviation beneath the skin over other reflex zones, for example the renal tract, could indicate changing pathology and has been used to detect impending or actual urinary tract infection (Tiran 2009).

STANDARDISING TREATMENTS

The procedure of the treatment session also varies between schools of thought. The Marquardt style of RZT teaches students to work on the reflex zones for individual body systems, working from one foot to the other and back as appropriate, which seems theoretically logical but could feel disjointed for the client. The Ingham method™ teaches students to treat the whole of the left foot first, then the whole of the right, although no rationalisation can be given for this, despite the fact that treating the left foot first effectively treats the latter half of the intestines before the first half. The common practice of working the reflex zones for the colon from the right foot to the left in the direction of peristalsis could also be considered debatable: would peristalsis be reversed if treatment was performed in the opposite direction? Clearly, the direction of peristalsis cannot be reversed by external forces, and contradicts the notion that the aim of reflexology is one of normalisation. Arguably, however, if reflexology has the power to have some clinical effect, for example treating constipation or normalising peristalsis, surely there must be some theoretical basis for this? Certainly, in clients with specific gastrointestinal symptoms or disease, working the gastrointestinal tract in a reverse direction could have detrimental effects and it would be inappropriate and unprofessional to go against currently accepted practice without further evidence to the contrary (Marquardt 2000; Tiran 2009).

This argument can be expanded to consider its application to working the reflex zones for the urinary system and whether it is essential to work in the direction of diuresis. Many generic reflexologists consider it normal practice to work the bladder reflex zone first, up the ureters and then into the kidneys, arguing that it facilitates improved access to the reflexes allowing thorough, systematic coverage, although why this theory does not apply in reverse has not been adequately explained to date (personal communications with reflexology practitioners and teachers). Practitioners of RZT dispute this traditional practice (Lett 2000; Marquardt 2000; Tiran 2009) and Tiran (2009) has clinical evidence of exacerbation of the effects of urinary tract infection in pregnant women through reflexology performed in the 'wrong' direction.

Some authorities also question the theory that dips or apparent 'emptiness' in a reflex zone may indicate an anatomical space, perhaps where an organ such as the appendix or uterus has been removed. Conversely, some experts have confirmed that it is possible to identify from the feet the absence of organs, or the presence of additional elements, for example a developing fetus, growing neoplasm or surgically implanted items such as an intrauterine contraceptive device (coil). Midwives who are experienced reflexologists can often determine, from the reflex zones on the feet, the position of the fetus, including diagnosis of a breech presentation in which the fetus presents bottom first, or indeed the dilatation of the cervix in labour by palpating the reflex zone for the cervix (not normally taught in basic training) (see Ch. 9 and Tiran 2009).

CONCLUSION

One of the greatest barriers to integration of reflexology within conventional healthcare is lack of consistency amongst therapists, due to the varied styles, techniques, traditions and 'rules' governing practice. However, the therapy is slowly, but surely evolving into a profession in its own right, and some of these inconsistencies are gradually being eroded to make way for a more standardised system of practice. To some reflexologists, this may be viewed as changing – or challenging – the status quo, whilst to others it may indicate a contemporary alteration to the issues which constantly influence any profession. Reflexology is a powerful therapy which deserves more than being seen merely as a pampering relaxation treatment. It has valid benefits for clients and patients and, in the future, may become an integral component of conventional healthcare, but this can only happen with a corporate approach, improved regulation, well-designed clinical research projects and enhanced status based on clear scientific guidelines. Further debate based, where possible, on contemporary evidence, will contribute to unification of the profession, and initiate new ways of working to provide a sound foundation from which education and practice can develop.

ACKNOWLEDGEMENTS

Clive O'Hara was a renowned and respected teacher and clinical practitioner in the world of reflexology in the UK. During more than 30 years of unbroken clinical practice he treated literally thousands of clients, a fact which undoubtedly qualified him as one of the leading experts in the field of complementary medicine. This chapter is dedicated to Clive who sadly passed away after a long illness in June 2008. It is based partly on Clive's original chapter in the first edition of *Clinical Reflexology* (2002) and on his more recent journal papers. The discussions in this chapter do not entirely reflect Clive's opinions, since practice advances and evolves, but we are certain that Clive would have felt honoured to have initiated such debate, and would have been delighted to have seen his beloved profession of reflexology moving ever forward to take its rightful place within the healthcare arena.

REFERENCES

American Heritage Dictionary of English Language Online, 2009. http://en.wikipedia.org/wiki/The_American_Heritage_Dictionary_of_the_English_Language.

Collins Online Dictionary, 2006. www.collinslanguage.com.

Gale, E., Hegarty, J.R., 2000. The use of touch in caring for people with learning disability. Br. J. Develop. Disabil. 46 (Part 2 (91)), 97–108.

Kohara, H., Miyauchi, T., Suehiro, Y., Ueoka, H., Takeyama, H., Morita, T., 2004. Combined modality treatment of aromatherapy, footsoak, and reflexology relieves fatigue in patients with cancer. J. Palliat. Med. 7 (6), 791–796.

Lett, A., 2000. Reflex zone therapy for health professionals. Churchill Livingstone, London.

Marquardt, H., 2000. Reflexotherapy of the feet. Thieme, Germany.

McVicar, A.J., Greenwood, C.R., Fewell, F., D'Arcy, V., Chandrasekharan, S., Alldridge, L.C., 2007. Evaluation of anxiety, salivary cortisol and melatonin secretion following reflexology treatment: a pilot study in healthy individuals. Complement. Ther. Clin. Pract. 13 (3), 137–145.

Merriam Webster Medical Dictionary, 2009. Last viewed online at www.merriam-webster.com/medical.

O'Hara, C., 2002. Challenging the 'rules' of reflexology. In: Mackereth, P., Tiran, D. (Eds.), Clinical reflexology: a guide for heatlhcare professionals. Elsevier, Edinburgh, Chapter 3, pp. 33–52.

O'Hara, C., 2006. Core curriculum for reflexology in the United Kingdom. Douglas Barry Publications, London.

O'Hara, C., 2008. A Step too Far? Clinical Reflexology News Issue 25, 4–10.

Oleson, T., Flocco, W., 1993. Randomized controlled study of premenstrual symptoms treated with ear, hand, and foot reflexology. Obstet. Gynaecol. 82 (6), 906–911.

Raz, I., Rosengarten, Y., Carasso, R., 2003. Correlation study between conventional medical diagnosis and the diagnosis by reflexology (non conventional). Harefuah 142 (8–9), 600–605, 646.

Siev-Ner, I., Gamus, D., Lerner-Geva, L., Achiron, A., 2003. Reflexology treatment relieves symptoms of multiple sclerosis: a randomized controlled study. Mult. Scler. 9 (4), 356–361.

Tiran, D., 2009. Reflexology for pregnancy and childbirth; a definitive guide for healthcare professionals. Elsevier Science, Edinburgh.

Tiran, D., Chummun, H., 2005. The physiological basis of reflexology and its use as a diagnostic tool. Complement. Ther. Clin. Pract. 11 (1), 58–64.

White, A.R., Williamson, J., Hart, A., Ernst, E., 2000. A blinded investigation into the accuracy of reflexology charts. Complement. Ther. Med. 8 (3), 166–172.

Williams, A.M., Davies, A., Griffiths, G., 2009. Facilitating comfort for hospitalized patients using non-pharmacological measures: preliminary development of clinical practice guidelines. Int. J. Nurs. Pract. 15 (3), 145–155.

Revisiting the 'rules' of reflexology

SECTION II
APPLICATIONS IN CLINICAL PRACTICE

INTRODUCTION

Section I explored key professional issues in contemporary reflexology practice. In Section II the focus is on the work of clinical reflexologists and how they have developed and integrated reflexology safely and skilfully within specialist practice. Innovative approaches are described using anonymous case studies to illustrate adaptations in application. As with the first edition, the areas of practice are not exhaustive but rather illustrate the diversity of health care situations from preconception to end of life care.

Chapter 8. Infertility – Denise Tiran. This chapter outlines the causes and conventional treatment of female and male infertility and considers how reflexology can be of use in supporting couples undergoing assisted conception. There is also some discussion of the legal, ethical and safety issues pertaining to reflexology practice for these clients.

Chapter 9. Pregnancy and childbirth – Denise Tiran. This chapter discusses the safety and efficacy of reflexology during pregnancy, childbirth and the postnatal period and attempts to dispel some of the myths surrounding treatment for these clients. The legal, ethical and professional issues, including the role and responsibilities of reflexologists, are also explored.

Chapter 10. Teaching parents to use reflexology – Liz Tipping, with a contribution from Jenny Gordon. This chapter explores the issues and benefits of teaching parents to provide reflexology and foot massage techniques for their children. The chapter explores styles of teaching and learning, and how to ensure that parental learning has taken place. There is a focus on understanding the baby's non-verbal communication to gain an understanding of when and how a reflexology treatment should be given.

Chapter 11. Adapted Reflextherapy for pain: an alternative physiotherapy approach – Gunnel Berry. This chapter explores an adaptation of reflex zone therapy, developed by the author, who has used it with her physiotherapy patients for many years. It is particularly effective for treating people suffering from chronic pain, notably those with neck trauma, such as a history of whiplash injury.

Chapter 12. Adapting reflexology for cancer care – Peter Mackereth and Anita Mehrez, with contributions from Julia Williams and Edwina Hodkinson. Reflexology is a popular intervention for patients and carers in cancer and palliative care settings. This chapter examines key issues in developing safe and skilled approaches to reflexology in this complex, diverse and challenging area of healthcare. Myths and concerns are examined and recommendations made, including creative techniques and adaptations to treatment delivery.

Chapter 13. Reflexology and withdrawal from addictive substances: a focus on smoking cessation – Paula Maycock and Peter Mackereth. The authors begin by briefly examining the broader issues of addiction, the effects of withdrawal and the role of reflexology, using a behavioural model to support the individual through the transition to embracing and sustaining a smoke-free state. Case studies are included to illustrate key issues and innovative approaches to clinical practice.

Chapter 14. Reflexology incorporating new techniques – Jill Norfolk, Jan Williamson and Denise Tiran. This chapter explores contemporary developments in reflexology, from experienced practitioners who have incorporated new techniques in practice, based on the theoretical principles of other complementary therapies. Three examples are given: foot-applied Bowen technique (Jill Norfolk), Precision reflexology (Jan Williamson) and structural reflex zone therapy (Denise Tiran).

Infertility

8

Denise Tiran

ABSTRACT

This chapter explores the growing issue of infertility and the ways in which reflexology may help couples who are having difficulty in conceiving. The causes and conventional medical methods of treating couples with infertility are considered. Precautions to reflexology are discussed and the use of reflexology, both for general relaxation to reduce stress levels, which can so often be a contributing factor, and as a treatment modality for specific causes, are also explored.

KEY WORDS

Infertility, subfertility, conception, ovulation, in vitro fertilisation, reflex zone therapy.

INTRODUCTION

Infertility – or more correctly, subfertility – is a problem for which couples increasingly seek complementary therapy treatment, with reflexology appearing to be amongst the most popular choices. Certainly, the relaxation response from reflexology may help to restore and maintain homeostasis in some

99

DOI: 10.1016/B978-0-7020-3167-0.00008-1

women, facilitating the body to normalise its functions and thus enabling them to become pregnant, and there is some interesting work being carried out in some centres in which reflexology is offered to women seeking specialist infertility treatment.

Subfertility is an extremely complex situation which, in some cases, cannot be remedied, and if the cause lies not with the woman but with her partner, treating the woman alone will not achieve pregnancy. However, many women seem convinced that reflexology is the answer to their difficulties and the media does nothing to dispel these convictions. It would, of course, be entirely unprofessional for practitioners of reflexology to claim to 'treat' infertility or to guarantee to facilitate conception. This may give false hope to couples, some of whom may never be able to have a baby naturally. The women, in particular, are desperate to conceive and may have been trying to become pregnant for many years. They are particularly vulnerable and – like some cancer patients – will try 'anything' for which there is a suggestion that it might be successful. Unfortunately, there are numerous online accounts in which therapists purport to have treated women who subsequently become pregnant, but this is not evidence that the reflexology treatment is effective in 'curing' the physiopathological cause of the infertility. Furthermore, some reflexologists who 'specialise' in treating women/couples for infertility have an extremely poor knowledge and understanding of the aetiology and predisposing factors of the condition, and of the conventional medical management, and it is imperative that the professional clinical reflexologist has addressed this before attempting to do more than simple relaxation treatments.

CAUSES

Couples are classified as subfertile after one year of having regular, unprotected sexual intercourse, with about one couple in six seeking professional help. The aetiology of infertility is a complex combination of physical, psychological and social factors and it is important to be aware of these.

The psychosocial reasons for an increase in infertility in recent years include high-pressure jobs, financial pressures, career women actively choosing to delay having children until their late thirties and divorces leading to second marriages at a later age. When a couple starts considering a family and the woman fails to become pregnant for some time despite having regular sex, there will be anxiety that there is a medical problem, compounded by feelings of guilt about their lifestyle and their delay in entering the pregnancy arena. Whilst a man continues to produce spermatozoa until much later in life, the number of eggs left in a woman in her thirties or even her forties is constantly declining with each subsequent menstrual cycle, and those that remain may not be accessible to the sperm for a variety of reasons. The reflexologist can be especially supportive in these cases, and a course of treatment may, for some couples, be all that is required to facilitate a reduction in stress hormones and a consequent rise in the hormones required for conception and pregnancy.

Some couples fail to conceive due to sexual difficulties. They may be having intercourse infrequently or not at the most appropriate stage of the woman's menstrual cycle, around ovulation. (This is fourteen days *before* the next menstrual period; women who have a long or overly short menstrual cycle have a variable length in the first – follicular – 'half' of the cycle, before ovulation occurs, but the second – luteal – phase is always fourteen days.) These difficulties may be due to social, domestic or occupational stressors, or sometimes lack of knowledge. For example, very occasionally, the relationship may not have been consummated, the couple either indulging in non-penetrative physical contact or inadvertent penetration of the anal sphincter or urethra, rather than the vaginal opening, usually through poor knowledge or embarrassment and inhibition. Psychological factors can also cause vaginismus in the woman, excessive muscular contraction due to fear, which prevents penile penetration. These women/couples need specialist psychosexual counselling; it is not within the remit of the reflexologist to attempt to treat them and the couple should be encouraged to return to their general practitioner for referral for appropriate treatment.

The physiopathological reasons for the condition may lie with either the female or the male partner, or a combination of both, but the nature of the problem often means that couples feel embarrassed to discuss it, since it is a very personal issue and because, due to societal expectations, people feel they have 'failed'. In women, the reasons for difficulty in conceiving can loosely be classified as failure to produce or release eggs, structural anatomical problems or pathological medical conditions. In men, the causes are almost always related to abnormalities of sperm production and/or release.

Problems with ovulation (release of an egg) may be due to hormonal imbalances in the hypothalamus, pituitary gland or ovaries and can be triggered by stress and lifestyle factors such as smoking, alcohol abuse, a history of sexually transmitted infections, excessive exercise, under- or overweight. Stress hormones, such as cortisol, adrenaline (epinephrine) and noradrenaline (norepinephrine) from the adrenal glands, are known to have adverse effects on the production of hormones necessary to conception, pregnancy and breast feeding, such as oxytocin (Uvnas-Moberg & Petersson 2005). Women need at least 17% of their body weight to be adipose tissue (fat), as oestrogens are stored in the fat; therefore, women who are severely anorexic almost always cease menstruating and ovulating. Conversely, obese women with a body mass index of 30 or above are more at risk of conditions such as severe diabetes mellitus, hypertension and other cardiovascular problems (Kelly-Weeder & O'Connor 2006), which in themselves can contribute to reduced fertility.

Other causes include polycystic ovary syndrome or excessive prolactin production from the pituitary gland. Polycystic ovary syndrome is the most common cause of failure to ovulate, and is due to multiple small cysts on the surface of the ovaries, together with a hormonal imbalance, leading to absent or irregular periods; characteristically women so affected may be of stocky, slightly masculine build and be considerably more hirsute than most women, although this is not universal. High circulating prolactin levels from conditions such as a benign pituitary tumour will suppress the oestrogen and progesterone required for development of the Graafian follicle and, therefore, ovulation is suppressed.

Some women are found to have blocked fallopian tubes, usually occurring as a result of previous infection (salpingitis), sometimes sexually acquired, as in the case of chlamydia. The incidence of this infection has become such a significant problem that all young people between the ages of 15 and 25 are now offered free chlamydia testing. Infection caused by this or other organisms can also affect the cervical mucus, thickening it so that the passage of sperm at intercourse becomes much more difficult; in addition some women develop anti-sperm antibodies, exacerbating the problem.

Uterine factors include fibroids, polyps and tumours, which are usually benign, or an abnormally shaped or positioned uterus. Growths on the wall of the uterus interfere with the endometrial lining which is shed during menstruation, and sometimes causes scarring; if conception does occur, this prevents implantation of the fertilised ovum. Endometriosis is another very common cause of infertility, in which tissue normally located within the uterus develops abnormally in other areas of the pelvis, such as the fallopian tubes, on the ovarian surface and in the pelvic cavity. It causes intense pain and discomfort during menstruation, while the development of scar tissue and adhesions in and around organs in the pelvic cavity will further compromise the chances of conception.

Occasionally, a genetic condition, such as Turner's syndrome, may mean that secondary sexual characteristics fail to appear and there is no ovarian activity. In mild cases the condition may not be diagnosed until the woman fails to conceive, although more commonly absence of the menarche (onset of menstruation at puberty) will have revealed it earlier. A few women with normal ovarian function may experience premature menopause, or the ovaries may be affected by disease, including cancer and the effects of treatments such as radio- or chemotherapy.

Immunological factors may also play a part and can contribute to unexplained infertility, repeated early miscarriages or failure of in vitro fertilisation. There is a chemical 'mismatch' between the mother's system and the embryo – which contains 'foreign' cells from the father – and the embryo fails to embed in the uterine lining or separates (miscarriage). Occasionally, this is seen as an 'allergy' to the partner which can cause pregnancy failure or complications (in some women, pre-eclampsia can also be caused by these immunological issues). If the woman changes her partner, for example, through divorce or separation, attempts at conception may be more – or less – successful with the new partner.

Male infertility is most commonly related to sperm abnormalities. Good-quality semen requires an adequate concentration of spermatozoa which are both normal in structure and sufficiently mobile to make the long arduous journey from the vagina, following ejaculation, to join with the ovum which has been released from the woman's ovary, usually somewhere within the fallopian tube. Spermatozoa consist of a head, body and tail, but in the normal 3 ml of ejaculate, with an average of 200–300 million sperms present, 30% may be abnormal, having either an absence or a duplication of one or more sections of the sperm.

Testicular problems may result in deficient production (i.e. number) of sperm; the causes may be associated with previous infections, stress, excessive alcohol consumption, smoking, recreational drug use or treatments for medical conditions, including pharmaceutical prescriptions or radiotherapy, but in many cases the cause is unknown. Certain occupations can contribute to reduced fertility, notably those involving chemicals, electricity or nuclear power. Occasionally, the reason may be hormonal, whilst any situation in which the local temperature around the testes is raised, for example a varicocele (dilated blood vessels) or simply wearing tight underpants, will also impede sperm production. Constantly using a mobile telephone, especially if it is kept in the trouser pocket between calls, has also been blamed for reduced sperm production, possibly because of the heat they generate or due to the electromagnetic radiation they emit (Agarwal et al. 2008).

If there is an obstruction in the vas deferens, or very occasionally an anatomical absence of the tube, semen production may be normal but there will be no sperm in the ejaculate; this condition can follow infections such as tuberculosis, or severe trauma to the testicles. In men who have undergone reversal of a vasectomy, anti-sperm antibodies may be produced which attack the sperm and inhibit their motility, so although the tubes are patent again, the chemistry remains alien to conception (Firth & Hurst 2005:606).

CONVENTIONAL MANAGEMENT OF INFERTILITY

When a couple eventually seeks medical help they may have been unsuccessfully trying to conceive for some considerable time and it will not have been an easy step to consult their doctor. The general practitioner may undertake some investigations but, if no treatable cause is readily found, usually refers couples who meet specific criteria for more specialist help. Women over the age of 35, with six to twelve months of infertility, or younger women who have been unsuccessful after a year of trying, will normally be referred to a specialist gynaecologist, particularly if hormone tests indicate ovarian failure, or there has been no response to drugs which aim to stimulate ovulation. If there have been negative results to some of the initial tests, such as semen analysis or a post-coital test, or if there is the possibility of disease in the pelvis or fallopian tubes, these couples will also be referred to the consultant.

A full medical history is taken from both partners and a general examination of the woman is performed. General lifestyle advice is given – diet, weight management, smoking, alcohol consumption, drug use (prescribed medication and recreational use) and dealing with stress. Blood is taken to test for rubella immunity and various hormone levels, and a pelvic ultrasound scan is performed to assess for structural abnormalities in the pelvis. The man is asked to produce a semen sample which is tested for the volume of semen, number and concentration of sperm, motility and normality of individual sperm and the white cell count, which may reveal infection.

These tests are fairly basic but if the cause is still not found, the couple undergoes more intrusive investigations, including a post-coital test, although the usefulness of this is now being questioned. The woman is asked to go to the clinic within six to eight hours of having intercourse (without washing), usually in the preovulatory phase of her menstrual cycle, and a sample of mucus is taken from the cervical canal and transferred to a slide to assess how the sperm reacts to the mucus. She may be required to have a hysterosalpingogram – an X-ray during which a dye is passed through the cervix, uterus and fallopian tubes to test for patency of the reproductive tract, especially the tubes. If no abnormality has yet been detected she may also need a laparoscopy under anaesthetic to view the pelvic organs directly and to detect problems such as tubal patency, endometriosis or pelvic adhesions from previous surgery, all of which may affect the woman's ability to conceive.

Unfortunately, the difficulties for couples attempting to conceive may be compounded by multiple factors, for example, the woman may have endometriosis and the partner may have a low sperm count. In themselves, these conditions do not always result in infertility, but when combined they seriously impair the chances of successful conception. The most common 'cause' of all is 'unexplained infertility' and these are, from a conventional medical perspective, the most difficult situations to remedy. An additional group of female patients includes those who manage to conceive yet who are unable to continue with the pregnancy, suffering multiple miscarriages. The causes of repeated pregnancy loss in the first trimester (three months) tend to be the same or similar to those for subfertility, but, of course, these women will be possibly even more psychologically and emotionally distressed, which does nothing to help the problem. Again, whilst it is the responsibility of the reflexologist not to overstep the boundaries of their practice by attempting to treat or 'cure' the situation, gentle empathetic support and relaxation reflexology can go a long way towards helping these couples to come to terms with their situation.

If a cause for the infertility is found it may be possible to treat the condition: medical treatment will always be dependent on the cause. Hormonal inadequacies in the woman are treated with drugs, and anatomical abnormalities may be treated with surgery; if the cause is a male factor, the man can be referred to an andrologist/endocrinologist to investigate further the causes of semen or hormonal abnormality.

Many women are prescribed drugs such as clomiphene (Clomid™) to stimulate ovulation. This is taken within the first five days of the menstrual cycle and continues for five days; ovulation should normally occur 5–13 days after taking the last tablet. If, after taking clomiphene for 6 months, ovulation has not occurred, a synthetic form of follicle-stimulating hormone is given by subcutaneous injection. Careful monitoring by the gynaecologist is required because excessive stimulation of the ovary is a not uncommon response; in some this may lead to multiple pregnancy, whilst in a minority, a serious complication can result in potentially life-threatening hyperstimulation syndrome.

If the woman fails to ovulate and conceive naturally following this, assisted reproduction may be considered, either through the NHS or privately. The general principles of assisted conception are: the stimulation of multiple follicles in the woman's ovary; preparation of a sperm sample if there is a reasonable concentration of normal sperm, with good motility; combining of the gametes to enhance the chance of fertilisation; re-implantation in the uterus of fertilised ova.

There are many different types of assisted reproduction, including intrauterine insemination in which an injection of washed sperm is inserted into the uterine cavity; use of sperm from a donor when the semen characteristics of the male partner are inadequate; and in vitro fertilisation in which the eggs are harvested from the woman and combined with the sperm in the laboratory. Contemporary techniques include blastocyst transfer, gamete intrafallopian transfer (GIFT) and zygote intrafallopian transfer (ZIFT), all of which involve re-implantation of the fertilised egg into the uterus, but differ with the stage of maturation of the fertilised egg in the laboratory prior to transfer. Micromanipulation is a technique which allows the embryologist to perform very precise surgical procedures on eggs and embryos, usually in cases where there is a risk of genetic diseases such as cystic fibrosis.

Intracytoplasmic sperm injection (ICSI) has revolutionised the treatment of male infertility, offering help to couples who previously would have had to rely on donor sperm. The initial procedure is the same as for in vitro fertilisation and other forms of assisted reproduction, but once in the laboratory a single sperm is injected into the centre of an egg. This is particularly valuable in cases where abnormality of sperm or a mismatch between the egg and the sperm prevent the sperm from penetrating the thick outer layer (zona pelucida) of the egg, which may be due to lack of the enzyme hyaluronidase.

Where the woman has been found unable to produce eggs or fails to achieve pregnancy using her own eggs, ovum donation, in which eggs from another woman are artificially impregnated with the partner's sperm, may be appropriate; alternatively, surrogacy, in which another woman agrees to incubate the pregnancy, may be considered. If no cause can be found or all medical treatment options have been exhausted, adoption may be considered or the couple may be offered counselling to help them come to terms with the fact that they will not have children.

GENERAL RELAXATION REFLEXOLOGY TO SUPPORT INFERTILE COUPLES

Reflexology practitioners wishing to support couples experiencing infertility problems must have a *thorough* understanding of the causes, manifestations and conventional treatment of the condition in general and its effects on the couple in particular. They should possess well-refined listening skills and must acknowledge their personal professional boundaries in respect of both the advice and information they give to couples and the level at which they stop listening and refer to someone with the appropriate counselling qualifications. There is also a need for therapists to recognise that they cannot *treat* the condition, but can have an important role to *support* the couple and to provide a therapeutic interaction which *may* facilitate enhanced homeostasis, hopefully leading to an improved chance of conception.

Many women turn to nutritional and other 'natural' methods of enhancing fertility. These are specialist areas of women's health which practitioners of nutritional therapy, naturopathy and herbal medicine have used very successfully to help couples achieve conception. However, reflexologists should be wary of incorporating these other disciplines into the advice they give couples. It is essential that they have been adequately and appropriately trained to use other therapies and can provide comprehensive advice based on contemporary research evidence; this must not conflict with Department of Health (DoH) guidelines on nutrition and diet. Similarly, it is not appropriate to combine therapies such as aromatherapy with reflexology unless the practitioner is fully aware of the chemical effects of the essential oils on the client(s), especially as there are many which should not be used during pregnancy or the preconceptional period.

Conversely, basic lifestyle advice can be offered as follows:

- Increase intake of: fruit, vegetables and salad; whole grains (brown rice, oats, wholemeal bread); phytoestrogens, including beans, lentils, chickpeas); oily foods (fish, nuts, seeds, pure vegetable oils); fibre-rich foods; fluid, especially water.
- Decrease intake of: saturated fat (dairy products, etc.); caffeine (coffee, tea, cola); sugar (beware 'hidden' sugars); additives, preservatives and chemicals, e.g. artificial sweeteners; red meat.
- Lifestyle factors: reduce alcohol consumption; stop smoking and recreational drug use; exercise for at least three sessions of 20 minutes weekly.
- Take folic acid or multivitamin supplements as recommended by the DoH for prepregnancy.

From a practical perspective, it is preferable for the reflexologist to treat both partners, at least until a specific cause has been found. Treatments may be given as often as weekly, time and financial constraints permitting, and the accumulative effects of ongoing therapy often prove to be beneficial in indirect ways, reducing fatigue and improving sleep (Lee & Sohng 2005), easing tension and anxiety (Quattrin et al. 2006) and encouraging a frame of mind in which the clients become receptive to making lifestyle changes, such as stopping smoking or altering the diet.

The relaxation aspect of reflexology is the most powerful tool that the practitioner can offer in these circumstances. It has been seen when treating patients with life-limiting illnesses that reflexology creates a space which allows them time to talk, to express concerns and worries and makes them receptive to advice and information (Mackereth et al. 2009). General touch therapies such as massage have been shown to reduce stress hormone levels and increase serotonin and other 'feel good' chemicals in a variety of patients (Field et al. 2005; Arroyo-Morales et al. 2008; Garner et al. 2008). Reflexology, even when self-administered, can contribute to reducing stress, anxiety and depression and enhancing the immune system (Lee 2006), whilst the therapeutic relationship between client and therapist can add to these effects. It may also be possible for the reflexologist to teach the couple how to treat each other in order to maintain the relaxation effect between treatments from the practitioner.

Regular contact with the practitioner can imbue the couple with a sense that something is 'being done' and that they are not alone, a factor which is frequently seen in couples who finally present for gynaecological treatment of infertility. Where the raised cortisol effects of anxiety and worry depress the reproductive hormone levels, preventing ovulation and fertilisation, these often spontaneously decline to more manageable levels once an appointment for specialist medical treatment has been given, and it is not unusual for women to arrive for their first appointment to find that they are actually pregnant! This could lead an unwise therapist to claim that reflexology has helped the woman to achieve conception, which does nothing to aid the credibility of reflexology amongst orthodox medical personnel. Care should also be taken by the therapist to preserve professional boundaries: it is relatively easy to become involved in such an emotionally charged situation and the reflexologist would be wise to engage in regular debriefing with a mentor. Conversely, the couple may come to rely on the reflexologist and to view him/her as the answer to their problems.

Emily was a 27-year-old woman who consulted the reflexologist because she was having trouble conceiving with her new partner. She had two children aged 12 and 8, and had been with Neil for 4 years. They had been having regular unprotected intercourse for two and a half years but Emily was still not pregnant and was now becoming increasingly stressed, dreading the appearance of every menstrual period. This was causing her to become very tearful and to demand sex frequently in an attempt to increase her chances of conception. The reflexologist was at pains to emphasise that there was no guarantee that the treatment would work because the cause of Emily's failure to become pregnant was not known and she had not yet consulted her general practitioner for a referral for specialist medical help. The reflexologist asked about Emily's medical and family history and, although Neil was not present, asked Emily what she knew about his medical history. There appeared to be nothing overtly pathologically significant in the medical history of either partner.

On examination of Emily's feet, the reflexologist noted an overall greyness and blotchiness to the skin which was not in keeping with Emily's generally rosy complexion; the shadowing on the feet was especially focused around the reflex zones for the heart and solar plexus areas. Emily had already acknowledged that she was stressed about not getting pregnant, but the therapist now asked her about major emotional upheavals in the last few years. Emily admitted that she had previously been in a very abusive relationship which had ended in a very acrimonious divorce shortly before she met Neil. The reflexologist, who also had a qualification in counselling, was able to ask Emily how she felt about her new relationship: Emily confessed that she loved Neil but found it difficult to trust him because of her previous experiences. She also recognised that her constant demands for sex were being counterproductive and that sex was becoming mechanical. Emily and the therapist spent some time during this first appointment talking about these issues, but as the therapist had not been approached specifically for counselling, she suggested that referral to one of her colleagues could be useful if Emily wished to work through them more deeply, and Emily welcomed this opportunity.

In the meantime, the reflexologist suggested that Emily should have a course of treatment aimed at relaxing her and reducing her stress levels. Emily found these weekly sessions very pleasant and became spontaneously motivated to consider other aspects of her lifestyle, including her diet, exercise and work situations. After 6 weeks, Emily felt much calmer and was not so obsessed every month about whether or not she started a menstrual period, her relationship with Neil had improved and they were, once again, enjoying their physical relationship. The therapist then suggested that Emily should invite Neil to come for treatment, to which she agreed and Neil had 3 weeks of general relaxation reflexology just after Emily's continuing treatments, which he enjoyed. At this point the therapist suggested that Emily and Neil should have some joint sessions in which they learned the skills of reflexology so that they could work on each other. After 2 more weeks the couple felt they could continue without the therapist's direct input (although she reassured them that they could call her at any time).

Six weeks later, after no further professional help, Emily telephoned the therapist to tell her that she had just had a positive pregnancy test – and was feeling extremely sick every morning. Emily returned for regular treatments throughout her pregnancy and 9 months later gave birth to a beautiful baby boy.

Related physical problems may also be treated with relaxation reflexology, which may have a direct impact on the chances of conception. Dysmenorrhoea (painful periods), which can occur in isolation, or in conjunction with problems such as endometriosis or fibroids, may be relieved by receiving gentle reflexology treatment in the early stage of the menstrual period, or immediately prior to menstruation. This can be particularly effective if the woman also suffers from premenstrual tension (Oleson & Flocco 1993) and she may be able to be taught self-administration or the therapist could teach the partner how to perform simple techniques (Kim et al. 2004). Whilst these are physiological conditions they are often exacerbated by psychological issues and, in this respect, a course of general reflexology treatment may be helpful.

PRECAUTIONS WHEN TREATING INFERTILE COUPLES

The most significant precaution which reflexologists must acknowledge relates to clients who are having specialist medical treatment for infertility. Reflexology can be relaxing and pave the way for couples undergoing the myriad intrusive and invasive tests and investigations. However, there are two stages when *no reflexology* should be performed: first, while the woman is taking drugs (by whatever route) aimed at stimulating ovulation, e.g. clomiphene; and secondly, when eggs which have been fertilised in the laboratory are re-implanted into the woman's uterus, until either pregnancy is confirmed and has become established (at least 8 weeks), or menstruation has occurred.

Furthermore, assisted reproduction such as in vitro fertilisation is expensive and some NHS trusts will fund only a single attempt to become pregnant, yet it takes an average of three attempts for most couples to conceive (personal communication with infertility consultant colleagues). In no way would the reflexologist wish to compromise a couple's one and only chance of pregnancy with NHS treatment by performing inappropriate therapy. The difficulty is in understanding precisely what constitutes 'inappropriate therapy', but since there is no real evidence to date of whether – or why – reflexology can effectively treat infertility, professional caution is justified. It is of real concern that some therapists mistakenly believe that no harm can come from continuing to treat women during the ovulation–stimulation phase or immediately after re-implantation of the eggs. If reflexology is effective enough to produce beneficial results in some people, by inference, inappropriate (or inaccurate) reflexology may do harm. Additionally, once the couple is unable to obtain free assisted conception on the NHS, they must pay for treatment privately, averaging about £4000 per cycle (attempt). It would be unethical to perform any reflexology treatment which may inadvertently interfere with medical treatment, however it is funded, but especially when couples are funding this themselves.

Given that the principal cause of female infertility is anovulation, relaxation reflexology can only facilitate ovum release if high stress hormone levels are responsible for suppressing the necessary release of oestrogen. If this failure to ovulate is due to a more pathological reason, reflexology may not be enough to trigger the Graafian follicle to mature, rupture and release the egg. Since most hormonal imbalances are due either to hypothalamic or pituitary malfunction, it would be reasonable to assume that stimulating these reflex zones might elicit the required response. However, this is an example of how important it is for the practitioner to understand the individual's personal circumstances, as some conditions cannot be treated and others may be worsened by the use of inappropriate reflexology techniques. For example, if a pituitary tumour is preventing follicular development (even if benign), overenthusiastic stimulation of the pituitary gland reflex zone could theoretically cause enlargement of the neoplasm, creating further suppression of pituitary hormones. Similarly, excessive stimulation of the ovarian reflex zones could, in women with polycystic ovary syndrome, induce excessive follicular development on the surface of the ovary which would elevate the abnormal luteinising hormone levels in the woman's blood, and cause a further increase in production of the male hormone, testosterone, complicating the clinical picture even more. Also, care should be taken when treating a woman with a uterine condition such as fibroids: stimulation of the reflex zone for the uterus should be avoided in order to prevent bleeding.

In other, albeit very rare, cases torrential postpartum haemorrhage in a previous labour can lead to a pituitary infarction (Sheehan's syndrome or pituitary necrosis), requiring lifelong hormone replacement (corticosteroids, oestrogen and growth hormones). No amount of reflexology treatment will enliven a part of the anterior pituitary gland which has, essentially, died.

A woman who is having difficulty in conceiving due to anorexia nervosa or bulimia and whose body mass index is excessively low (below 16), cannot be treated adequately with reflexology until she has gained weight, since adipose tissue (fat) assists in converting androgens to the oestrogens required to stimulate ovulation. Furthermore, the often severe psychological problems suffered by women who are anorexic mean that these clients are outside the remit of most therapists unless they have specialist qualifications in counselling.

Where the woman has been found to have blocked fallopian tubes due to salpingitis (direct infection in the tubes), or from indirect infection which has descended from other organs such as the appendix, it is unlikely that natural conception can occur. However, if one or both tubes are damaged but not entirely blocked (this may not have been clinically confirmed) *gentle* reflexology over the reflex zones for the ovaries, tubes, pelvic lymphatics and uterus theoretically may help to restore the anatomy to a healthier condition. It is *absolutely imperative* that the reproductive tract reflex zones are worked from the ovary towards the uterus and *not* in the reverse direction, as any residual infection could be spread further. Women with a history of previous salpingitis who have not yet accessed specialist medical care for their infertility should be advised to request a blood test for sexually transmitted infections, notably chlamydia, from their general practitioner.

If the woman has severe endometriosis there may be anatomical disruption due to the presence of scar tissue, as well as cysts on the ovaries which prevent ovulation from occurring. Although, as has been mentioned, the woman may appreciate the pain-relieving effects of relaxation reflexology, extreme care should be taken not to overstimulate the area of the pelvic reflex zones, as well as those for the abdominal organs. Other anatomical deviations in the uterus, such as a bicornuate or septate uterus (two-horned or completely divided in two, respectively), are associated with a high risk of miscarriage in the event of conception occurring, and any female client known to have this abnormality should be treated extremely carefully.

If there is any doubt about whether or not a client may be pregnant she should be treated as if she *is* pregnant (see Ch. 9 on pregnancy and childbirth). The reflexologist who believes the client may be pregnant should *in no way* stimulate or sedate the ovaries, uterus or pituitary gland as this may adversely affect continuation of a tentative pregnancy. Also it is highly inappropriate for a therapist to make any claims, from an examination of the feet, that a woman may or may not be pregnant – the only firm factual knowledge on which the woman or her therapist can rely is that the client is *not* pregnant because she is menstruating!

REFLEX ZONE THERAPY FOR SPECIFIC INDICATIONS RELATED TO INFERTILITY

Reflex zone therapy (RZT) is a specific type of reflexology for clinical practice, in which the body and the feet are divided into longitudinal and horizontal zones, with some variations in the reflex zones (points) and maps (charts); treatment aims to facilitate recognition of disordered foot zones, to relieve symptoms of physiopathological conditions and to prevent further complications. It could be argued to be a more reductionist form of reflexology, since some zones are treated in isolation in order to elicit a therapeutic response using various manual compression techniques, some stimulating and some sedating, with the aim of rebalancing homeostasis and triggering the body's innate self-healing capacity (see Tiran 2010).

If the true cause of a couple's infertility has been confirmed it may be possible for a suitably trained reflex zone therapist to provide treatment aimed at resolving or reducing the impact of the cause. For example, appropriate stimulation of the relevant reflex zones can initiate or increase hormonal

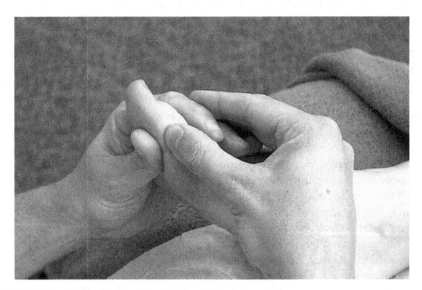

FIG. 8.1 Practitioner working the neck area. *Photo courtesy of Katie Spruce BA (Hons), medical photographer, Christie Hospital NHS Trust, with permission.*

production, but this should only be undertaken by practitioners with a thorough knowledge of hormone physiology and who are able to apply this knowledge to the individual's physiology. RZT is, however, a specialist clinical field and it is not the purpose of this book to cover specific treatments in depth.

RESEARCH EVIDENCE

To date, there is *no evidence* from studies of good calibre to demonstrate that reflexology treats infertility.

Although there has been one previous study, of dubious methodology, in which 108 women received non-specified reflexology for infertility (Eriksen 1994), the only contemporary study was undertaken in Devon (Holt et al. 2008), but unfortunately the validity of the study is suspect. A two-year trial investigated whether or not receiving reflexology increased conception in anovulatory women, randomised to receive either 'true' reflexology or 'sham' reflexology in the form of foot massage. It is necessary to consider whether the treatment was purely a relaxation treatment, which could be effective in the same way as other touch therapies such as massage, or whether it incorporated specific techniques, as in reflex zone therapy, which would need to address the causative factors and would be difficult to standardise in terms of research methodology. The fact that treatments were performed by a single practitioner further compromised the methodology as the therapeutic interaction could have been instrumental in reducing stress levels and potentially improving conception rates. In addition, the use of 'sham' reflexology involving foot massage is not sufficiently different from foot reflexology to be truly valid in terms of the effects of touch. Sadly, preliminary work by the research team suggests that, while randomisation and blinding of subjects is possible, there was no statistically significant increase in ovulation in those receiving true reflexology, and that 'sham' reflexology may have some non-specified effects on infertile women, although the researchers recognise that the initial study was very small (Holt et al. 2008).

CONCLUSION

It is irresponsible for practitioners to make spurious and unfounded claims that reflexology can 'treat' infertility, particularly when the emphasis is on an increasing use of evidence to support practice. However, despite the lack of any real evidence to demonstrate that reflexology is effective in dealing with the direct physiopathological causes of subfertility, we do have evidence of its benefits in relieving stress and enhancing the neurochemical antecedents which contribute to a couple's ability to conceive. Touch alone is a powerful modality, especially when combined with the psychoemotional impact of a trusting and empathetic relationship with the therapist. Indeed, the placebo effect can also be a therapeutic action in its own right, in this case potentially increasing self-confidence and feelings of self-worth to levels which improve the homeostatic balance so that the client's body, mind and spirit become receptive to a culmination of the factors which assist in achieving – and maintaining – a pregnancy. The reflexologist is in a privileged and powerful position to engage with these clients, but must also acknowledge the responsibilities which come with that relationship.

RECOMMENDATIONS FOR PRACTICE

- Develop a theoretical understanding of the causes, effects and medical treatments of infertility.
- Never make claims guaranteeing to treat the condition.
- If the cause is unknown, treatment should be primarily for relaxation.
- Reflex zone therapy to treat the cause should only be performed by practitioners who have a thorough understanding of the problem, and only after consultation with the doctor.
- Do *not* perform reflexology during the time when the woman is taking drugs to stimulate ovulation, or once artificially fertilised ova (eggs) have been re-implanted into the uterus until pregnancy has been confirmed and is well established (at least 8 weeks).

REFERENCES

Agarwal, A., Deepinder, F., Sharma, R.K., Ranga, G., Li, J., 2008. Effect of cell phone usage on semen analysis in men attending infertility clinic: an observational study. Fertil. Steril. 89 (1), 124–128.

Arroyo-Morales, M., Olea, N., Martínez, M.M., Hidalgo-Lozano, A., Ruiz-Rodríguez, C., Díaz-Rodríguez, L., 2008. Psychophysiological effects of massage-myofascial release after exercise: a randomized sham-control study. J. Altern. Complement. Med. 14 (10), 1223–1229.

Eriksen, L., 1994. Has reflexology an effect on infertility? FDZ Research Committee, Denmark. Viewed at www.reflexologyresearch.net/ReflexologyInfertilityResearch.shtml.

Field, T., Hernandez-Reif, M., Diego, M., Schanberg, S., Kuhn, C., 2005. Cortisol decreases and serotonin and dopamine increase following massage therapy. Int. J. Neurosci. 115 (10), 1397–1413.

Firth, H.V., Hurst, J.A., 2005. Oxford desk reference clinical genetics. Oxford University Press, Oxford.

Garner, B., Phillips, L.J., Schmidt, H.M., Markulev, C., O'Connor, J., Wood, S.J., et al., 2008. Pilot study evaluating the effect of massage therapy on stress, anxiety and aggression in a young adult psychiatric inpatient unit. Aust. N. Z. J. Psychiatry 42 (5), 414–422.

Holt, J., Lord, J., Acharya, U., White, A., O'Neill, N., Shaw, S., et al., 2008. The effectiveness of foot reflexology in inducing ovulation: a sham-controlled randomized trial. 91 (6), 2514–2519.

Kelly-Weeder, S., O'Connor, A., 2006. Modifiable risk factors for impaired fertility in women: what nurse practitioners need to know. J. Am. Acad. Nurse Pract. 18 (6), 268–276.

Kim, Y.S., Kim, M.Z., Jeong, I.S., 2004. The effect of self-foot reflexology on the relief of premenstrual syndrome and dysmenorrhea in high school girls. Taehan Kanho Hakhoe Chi 34 (5), 801–808.

Lee, Y.M., 2006. Effect of self-foot reflexology massage on depression, stress responses and immune functions of middle aged women. Taehan Kanho Hakhoe Chi 36 (1), 179–188.

Lee, Y.M., Sohng, K.Y., 2005. The effects of foot reflexology on fatigue and insomnia in patients suffering from coal workers' pneumoconiosis. Taehan Kanho Hakhoe Chi 35 (7), 1221–1228.

Mackereth, P.A., Booth, K., Hillier, V.F., Caress, A.L., 2009. What do people talk about during reflexology? Analysis of worries and concerns expressed during sessions for patients with multiple sclerosis. Complement. Ther. Clin. Pract. 15 (2), 85–90.

Oleson, T., Flocco, W., 1993. Randomized controlled study of premenstrual symptoms treated with ear, hand, and foot reflexology. Obstet. Gynecol. 82 (6), 906–911.

Quattrin, R., Zanini, A., Buchini, S., Turello, D., Annunziata, M.A., Vidotti, C., et al., 2006. Use of reflexology foot massage to reduce anxiety in hospitalized cancer patients in chemotherapy treatment: methodology and outcomes. J. Nurs. Manag. 14 (2), 96–105.

Tiran, D., 2010. Reflexology for pregnancy and childbirth: a definitive text for healthcare professionals. Elsevier, Edinburgh.

Uvnas-Moberg, K., Petersson, M., 2005. Oxytocin, a mediator of anti-stress, well-being, social interaction, growth and healing. Z. Psychosom. Med. Psychother. 51 (1), 57–80.

FURTHER READING

Andrews, G. (Ed.), 2005. Women's sexual health, third ed. Elsevier, Edinburgh.

USEFUL RESOURCES

www.infertilitynetworkuk.com – support network providing information and support to those affected by infertility.

www.foresight-preconception.org.uk – association for promotion of preconception care.

Pregnancy and childbirth

9

Denise Tiran

ABSTRACT

Traditionally, it has been considered by many reflexologists that it is unsafe to treat pregnant women, particularly in the first 3 months when there is an increased risk of miscarriage, and many of the early reflexology textbooks perpetuated this notion. However, reflexology can be a wonderfully relaxing therapy for expectant mothers and can be useful as a means of treating symptoms of pregnancy and easing childbirth, and many women now specifically seek out reflexology. However, therapists should ensure that they are able to treat mothers and their unborn babies safely, by considering the precautions, contraindications and effects of reflexology at this time.

KEY WORDS

Pregnancy, childbirth, maternity care, safety, professional responsibilities.

© 2011 Elsevier Ltd. All rights reserved.
DOI: 10.1016/B978-0-7020-3167-0.00009-3

BENEFITS OF REFLEXOLOGY IN PREGNANCY AND CHILDBIRTH

Reflexology has become very popular amongst expectant mothers in recent years, as well as for couples having difficulty with conceiving (see Ch. 8). Many pregnant women actively seek treatment at this time, usually for general relaxation. Some may have had reflexology prior to conception, whilst others request treatment to ease specific pregnancy discomforts. One of the factors welcomed by expectant mothers is the chance to develop a relationship with a professional therapist, especially as there is a severe shortage of some 5000 midwives in the UK. This means that, in conventional maternity care, emphasis is placed on monitoring and treating the mother's physical condition, whilst her myriad questions and concerns may go unanswered.

Reflexology during pregnancy appears to have profound benefits, although whether this is due to the physical effects of reflexology, the therapeutic value of human touch, or the psychological effects of the client–therapist interaction is debatable. Relaxation reflexology allows the mother to have time for herself, and the ongoing physical and emotional effects of the treatment assist in preparing her for the birth. When physical discomforts occur during the pregnancy, the reflexologist may then be able to use specific techniques to treat the mother for problems such as nausea, backache, sciatica, headaches, carpal tunnel syndrome and constipation. Increasingly too, mothers are requesting practitioners to accompany them during labour, to provide pain relief and emotional support and to act as their advocate by liaising with conventional maternity professionals. Some therapists may already work as doulas (lay birth supporters) whereas others may develop a close relationship with a particular client and wish to support her throughout the childbearing process. Postnatally, reflexology can aid adaptation to parenthood, facilitate breast feeding (or cessation of lactation) and may prevent or reduce the severity of postnatal depression.

LEGAL AND PROFESSIONAL ISSUES

Many expectant mothers like to use a range of complementary therapies or natural remedies, such as massage, aromatherapy, and herbal or homeopathic medicines, although there is a relatively limited amount of research evidence on the safety and effectiveness of reflexology in particular, as opposed to manual therapies in general. This apparent lack of evidence has led the National Institute for Health and Clinical Excellence (NICE) to recommend health professionals to discourage women from using complementary therapies during pregnancy or birth (National Collaborating Centre 2008). This is not particularly helpful, nor entirely accurate, but it may mean that some conventional maternity care providers (midwives and doctors) are reluctant to condone women's alternative treatments by independent therapists. Fortunately, however, this situation is slowly changing, as many midwives now use manual therapies in their own practice, although availability remains slightly ad hoc (Williams & Mitchell 2007). Many maternity units now offer reflexology, massage, aromatherapy or shiatsu (Dhany 2008; Lythgoe & Metcalfe 2008; Mitchell & Allen 2008), particularly in response to the need to focus on keeping birth normal to avoid medical interventions and reduce an escalating national

Caesarean section rate, which is approaching 25%. Indeed, the Department of Health document, *Maternity Matters* (2007), now appears committed to the concept of providing a 'full range of birthing choices', including complementary therapies to ease pain in labour.

TRAINING AND CONTINUING PROFESSIONAL DEVELOPMENT

Reflexologists who are not qualified midwives or doctors must recognise the limitations of their own professional accountability. Those who wish to specialise in treating pregnant women must have a thorough understanding of pregnancy physiology, embryonic and fetal development, potential maternal and fetal pathology (see Case Study 9.1), the current maternity services and the role and responsibilities of the practitioner, especially when working within an NHS maternity unit.

CASE STUDY 9.1 LAURA

Laura was receiving regular reflexology from the complementary therapy (CT) midwife to keep her blood pressure within normal limits, as it had been very high in her previous pregnancy. At her 32-week appointment she arrived looking generally unwell, stating that her ankles had been very swollen 4 days before and that she had had a headache, but had done nothing about it. Her headache persisted and her ankles remained very oedematous. On questioning, Laura said she felt sick, had visual disturbance and right-sided epigastric pain, all symptoms of fulminating pre-eclampsia. The CT midwife took her blood pressure, which was extremely high, and then went to confer with a colleague regarding relevant blood tests to exclude further complications. On her return Laura said she felt a sudden pounding behind her eyes, and her skin had turned grey. The midwife became alarmed, assessing Laura as possibly about to have an eclamptic fit, and rushed to transfer her to the delivery suite. On investigation, it transpired that Laura had a severe urinary tract infection that was mimicking impending eclampsia. This was treated immediately by the medical staff to prevent preterm labour commencing, but Laura's blood pressure did not respond and it was decided to deliver the baby that night by Caesarean section.

The point at issue here is not that the midwife was mistaken in her diagnosis but that, taking into account the speed with which Laura's condition deteriorated, the midwife was alert enough to act swiftly on the assumption of one of the most serious complications of pregnancy. This demonstrates the need to understand fully the pathophysiology of pregnancy and to work in conjunction with the conventional maternity services.

Whilst core curricula for reflexology training programmes now recommend students to have an introduction to the treatment of pregnant women (O'Hara 2007), this is rarely sufficient to engender confidence in the practitioner. It would be wise for those intending to treat pregnant women to have undertaken continuing professional development to ensure that they can apply generic reflexology principles to the specific physiopathology of pregnancy and that they have a thorough understanding of the maternity services. This should also include knowledge of the first aid treatment that may be necessary in a variety of situations. Examples include: precipitate labour (completed in under 2 hours); antepartum haemorrhage (vaginal bleeding after 28 weeks' gestation); eclamptic fit (a serious and sometimes fatal consequence of pre-eclampsia, the pregnancy-specific high blood pressure syndrome); or cord prolapse following spontaneous rupture of the membranes (in which the umbilical cord drops below the level of the baby's head, leading to oxygen deprivation and possible fetal death).

Adequate listening skills are essential, as pregnant women frequently ask for advice and reassurance, but this may sometimes mask a subconscious request for more focused help, for example with sexual problems in pregnancy or domestic violence issues. It is fundamental to good practice that the reflexologist is adequately prepared to answer even the most basic of questions: with antenatal clients this presumes a thorough working knowledge of contemporary, evidence-based information on aspects such as diet and lifestyle, specifically related to pregnancy. It is not, for example, appropriate to attempt to advise women on dietary issues based on inadequate or out-of-date knowledge, and practitioners should be aware of the current Department of Health guidelines on healthy eating (see www.dh.gov.uk).

Practitioners need also to maintain continual updating in both their reflexology skills *and* in current trends in maternity care which are pertinent to their work. Occasionally, reflexologists incorporate elements of other therapies, such as basic acupressure point stimulation or massage with aromatherapy oils alongside their main therapy, but it is *vital* to understand fully the application of these additional therapies to pregnant and childbearing women and the potential for interaction between therapies. For example, some practitioners may incorporate essential oils in their reflexology treatment, but many of these are contraindicated during pregnancy and childbirth (see Tiran 2000), as are numerous herbal remedies (Chuang et al. 2006), while stimulation of certain acupressure points is prohibited during pregnancy as this may trigger contractions, causing preterm labour. All practitioners, both conventional and complementary, should be able to justify their actions, supported by research-based evidence where available. It is unprofessional and potentially professionally suicidal, especially in this age of litigation, to act without full knowledge, understanding and experience of the therapies and the client group.

RECORDS AND CONFIDENTIALITY

Midwives and doctors are legally required to retain maternity notes for 25 years. This is because, under the Congenital Disabilities (Civil Liability) Act of 1976, any claim for negligence can be taken to court by a child allegedly damaged by care during birth, for up to 25 years after the event. There is an expectation that childbirth in the Western world of the twenty-first century is safe: the death of a baby – or occasionally a mother – is so much more emotive than the death of someone who is elderly or seriously ill. Cases involving alleged maternity negligence account for almost 60% of claims dealt with by the NHS Litigation Authority and over £1 billion has been paid in compensation for maternity cases since 2001 (Independent newspaper 4-3-07).

Although there is no legal obligation on the part of therapists to retain their records for the full 25 years, it may be wise to do so, as any professional involved in the mother's care may be called to give evidence and it would be extremely difficult to remember details after so long a period of time. If the therapist feels unable to store all the documentation, she or he can request that notes on pregnant clients are sent to the maternity unit responsible for the mother's care, to be inserted into the individual mother's conventional maternity records. It is not permissible for the reflexologist to write in the conventional maternity notes when recording treatments but a copy of the reflexology record could be inserted in the back of these notes. This provides a reasonable means of communication between the therapist and the midwife caring for the mother, although more direct communication is wise on occasions. Since the potential for litigation is high when treating pregnant and/or labouring women, it is also important to ensure that the therapist has adequate and appropriate indemnity insurance cover; some companies providing insurance for complementary therapies do not cover the treatment of pregnant or labouring mothers.

Midwives are the principal maternity care providers, caring for women during pregnancy and for up to 28 days after delivery, and acting as the lead professional for approximately 70% of births. Midwives are the experts in caring for women with normal pregnancies and are trained to recognise when complications are developing, at which point they refer the mother to an obstetrician. Obstetricians are doctors who specialise in caring for women with problems in pregnancy and labour. If all is well, a mother does not need to consult a doctor at all, although a few choose to receive antenatal care from their general practitioner.

It is illegal for anyone other than a midwife or doctor, or one in training under supervision, to take sole responsibility for the care of expectant and labouring women, except in an emergency. There are, of course, occasional situations in which a baby arrives unexpectedly quickly and the mother will be glad of any help available. However, it is illegal for someone to plan to attend a mother during childbirth without having the requisite qualifications; indeed, there have been cases involving prosecution of men attending their partners during delivery, without the midwife being present. This is a growing contemporary problem, fuelled by public dissatisfaction with the maternity services, a severe shortage of midwives in some areas of the country and women's desire for more control over the childbearing experience. A new trend from the USA, 'unassisted birth' or 'free-birthing', means that some women are actively choosing to labour without professional support.

The reflexologist should therefore determine whether the mother is booked for conventional maternity care, either with the NHS or privately, with a midwife or a doctor. One way of confirming this is to ask to see the mother's maternity notes, which she keeps with her for the duration of the childbearing episode. If she is unable to produce these on demand, especially in later pregnancy as the birth approaches, the therapist may be alerted to the possibility that the mother intends to labour without professional help. In this case he or she should decline to provide maternity reflexology in order to protect his or her professional status.

Confidentiality is, of course, important in respect of all clients. However, it is very easy when caring for pregnant women to forget the need for discretion, especially as the outcome is usually so positive and exciting. Reflexologists should take extra care that colleagues with whom they discuss cases are only given information on a 'need to know' basis. When home visits are provided, consideration should be given to the mother who does not wish her neighbours to know that she is pregnant, especially in the early weeks – this may, for example, require a coat to be worn over the uniform, if one is worn.

Therapists intending to offer their services within an NHS maternity unit will need to have a Criminal Records Bureau check prior to working with pregnant women and their babies. Even those who do not enter the maternity unit but who choose to treat pregnant women and their babies would be wise to obtain this check privately. Some NHS trusts may also request reflexologists to sign an indemnity form, confirming that they have personal professional indemnity insurance cover and that, in the event of a case for negligence, they will not attempt to use the trust's vicarious liability cover (which only applies to employees of the trust). Further, practitioners may be asked to sign that they acknowledge that the midwife and/or doctor retains overall responsibility for the mother's care and that they agree to 'step back' if it is deemed no longer suitable for a mother to receive reflexology; this applies particularly to labour care. On occasions, this request may be made by the midwife, perhaps because of her lack of understanding of the therapy, even though the reflexologist may feel she or he still has a part to play. It is not appropriate to debate the situation at length in front of the labouring mother at this time, but a post-birth 'debriefing' between the two professionals can be helpful for both the midwife and the therapist and may strengthen their relationship for the future.

MATERNITY CARE IN THE UK

Antenatal care may be provided in the home, the GP's surgery or health centre and in the hospital maternity unit, both on the NHS and privately: some women choose to contract with an independent midwife whom they pay direct (average cost for pregnancy, labour and postnatal care is about £3500, rising to £6000 in London). Women may give birth at home (currently approximately 3–5% in most areas), in a midwife-led, low-risk birthing unit or in the consultant-led obstetric unit (maternity unit), depending on their choice, maternal and fetal health and local availability.

The midwife provides holistic woman-centred care, attending to her physiological, psychological, emotional and social needs, offering advice and education to prepare her for the birth and for parenthood, monitoring of maternal and fetal well-being and treatment or referral for specialist tests, investigations or management of her condition as necessary. In the event that the mother develops complications requiring medical care, the midwife continues to have a legal obligation alongside the doctor for the mother's ongoing care, from pregnancy, through to 28 days after delivery. Although midwives are qualified to provide the full range of care from conception to the postnatal period, many specialise in aspects such as ultrasound scanning, parent education, complementary therapies, or in caring for women with specific medical conditions including HIV/AIDS or sickle cell disease, or social circumstances such as domestic violence, teenagers or particular ethnic groups. During pregnancy, women have an initial appointment with the midwife in which a full medical, social and lifestyle history is taken and arrangements are made for necessary antenatal care and for delivery. Periodic appointments with the midwife, initially monthly, then fortnightly and weekly as the birth approaches, enable the maternal and fetal conditions to be monitored and the mother's questions to be answered, although in reality, appointments are usually short, which precludes in-depth discussion unless the midwife is alerted to a serious need.

RISKS OF REFLEXOLOGY IN PREGNANCY AND CHILDBIRTH

There has been much controversy about whether reflexology is safe for pregnant women, with students being taught to refrain from treating them during the first trimester, and the majority of traditional textbooks support this. However, practitioners can be reassured that reflexology, administered *correctly and appropriately*, in line with recognised professional boundaries, will not cause miscarriage, preterm labour, fetal malformations, vaginal bleeding or other pregnancy complications. This caution appears to be more a self-protective mechanism for the profession rather than being based on any research evidence, but many reflexologists are understandably cautious when treating pregnant women, with some declining to treat them at all. In any case, therapists may have been treating women prior to conception who then wish to continue with treatment. Some women will actively choose not to inform anyone of their suspected pregnancy until it has become established, so reflexologists may, in fact, be treating pregnant women without knowing it. This suggests that therapists should consider the theoretical possibility of pregnancy in all sexually active female clients of reproductive age (14–50), and should make it part of their normal practice to ask all female clients the date of the last menstrual period at each appointment. If there is any doubt about the date of the last menstrual period, or if a client is actively trying to conceive, they should be treated *as if* they are pregnant.

Conversely, some practitioners believe that, because reflexology is a natural therapy and pregnancy is a normal physiological event, no harm can come from treating women at this time. However, reflexology is a powerful tool that can have very beneficial effects, but by inference, if it is administered without due regard for safety, it could lead to undesired reactions. Loss of a pregnancy in the first trimester occurs naturally in 25% of pregnancies, as a result of physiopathological or psychological factors; there is no research evidence available to confirm or deny that reflexology could cause abortion. Sadly, women who suffer miscarriage often strive to find a reason for it and may, in the absence of any known aetiology, attribute their loss to the reflexology treatments they have received. It is therefore wise to act with caution, especially during the first trimester, the commonest time for miscarriage to occur, and particularly if the therapist is not a midwife. It is also necessary to acknowledge that any reflexology performed during pregnancy must take account of the fact that both the client *and* the fetus are being treated.

Reflexology performed with due caution, primarily for general relaxation, will do no harm and might, of course, be very beneficial. However, when practitioners are requested to provide treatment which encompasses specific techniques for easing pregnancy or postnatal discomforts or for aiding progress and comfort in labour, it is *absolutely imperative* that the reflexologist understands the mechanism of the treatment she or he administers and the physiopathology of the mother's condition. For example, when treating women with 'morning sickness' it is necessary to attempt to determine the cause of the symptoms and then to decide on the most appropriate course of action. Whilst nausea and vomiting in pregnancy is a common problem, affecting almost 90% of mothers, and normally attributed to hormonal fluctuations, it may be due also to thyroid deficiency or to gastrointestinal infection (Tiran 2004). It would therefore be inappropriate to overstimulate the reflex point for the thyroid gland, or to sedate the stomach or intestinal points, respectively, without understanding the precise pathology. Another common complaint in later pregnancy is backache, and it is easy to assume that this is the normal musculoskeletal backache related to increasing weight and lumbar lordosis (curvature due to hormonal effects), yet it may actually indicate a complication such as a urinary tract infection which, if left untreated, can trigger premature labour. Similarly, in labour, if the placenta is slow to deliver after the birth of the baby, it is essential to know (from the midwife) what precisely has occurred (and to understand the implications of this), as incorrect treatment could precipitate a torrential haemorrhage, which could be fatal in some cases. The fundamental issue is that reflexologists must be able to apply the principles of their therapy to the precise physiology of the individual mother's condition.

CONTRAINDICATIONS AND PRECAUTIONS

Pregnancy is a normal physiological condition for the majority of expectant mothers and reflexology at this time is both pleasurable and safe when undertaken by a qualified therapist experienced in treating this particular client group. Reflexologists who are in any doubt regarding the appropriateness of treating a particular client should refrain from doing so unless and until they have sought the relevant advice from the mother's midwife. There are, however, some situations in which reflexology should be avoided and others in which caution should be employed (Box 9.1).

A mother with a history of miscarriage, especially if she has had more than one, should receive only very gentle basic relaxation treatment – or even just simple foot massage – until after the gestation at which the latest miscarriage occurred. In some of these women it may be wise to delay any real treatment until after about 16 weeks' gestation, although the relaxation which the mother could gain from careful reflexology may be beneficial in itself. It is therefore necessary for the therapist to make an individual decision based on the mother's personal history and circumstances, before offering any treatment. *Any* vaginal bleeding in later pregnancy (after the first trimester) is abnormal and usually originates from partial separation of the placenta – either a placenta that is situated normally in the top part of the uterus (placental abruption) or a placenta that is embedded low down in the uterus, sometimes lying across the cervix and being incompatible with a normal vaginal delivery (placenta praevia). No reflexology should be performed whilst bleeding is active, and once it has subsided the reflexologist should consult the mother's midwife to ascertain whether it is appropriate or not to resume treatment.

Similarly, if a mother has a history of going into labour prematurely in previous pregnancies, she should not be treated around this time (usually between 28 and 34 weeks' gestation) except with gentle foot massage as opposed to specific reflexology techniques, although it is usually permissible to treat her after 34 weeks. Mothers expecting twins can be treated carefully, but it is necessary to consult the mother's obstetrician if a woman expecting triplets or quadruplets requests treatment, as the risk of complications increases with the number of fetuses.

Although reflexology has been shown to have a good effect in reducing blood pressure (Ejindu 2007), the therapist should identify those women with mild hypertension in pregnancy who may respond well to treatment, and those with more severe hypertension verging on serious pre-eclampsia, in whom treatment is inappropriate. Oedematous ankles are normal in pregnancy, but if the swelling extends to the knees and the mother exhibits oedema elsewhere such as in her face and fingers, together with a sudden weight increase, suggesting abdominal oedema, her condition may be deteriorating. Whilst she feels well in the early stages of the disease, any symptoms such as headache in late pregnancy, visual disturbance, and nausea and pain in the right side below the diaphragm are indicators of a worsening of pre-eclampsia which can lead to the extremely serious, potentially fatal situation in which the mother has epileptic-type fits (eclampsia). Therefore the reflexologist should assess the mother at each appointment to ensure that she remains fit and well and that there has been no significant change since the last visit.

Mothers with certain medical conditions should also not be treated during pregnancy, as the medical condition may adversely affect the pregnancy or vice versa. Sometimes a pre-existing condition such as hypertension, diabetes mellitus, epilepsy or cardiac disease worsens considerably during pregnancy and can, in the case of epilepsy and diabetes, become very unstable. They may also compromise the prognosis or progress of the pregnancy, either by increasing the risk of miscarriage, preterm labour or pregnancy-induced problems such as pre-eclampsia, or by adversely affecting fetal development, growth or well-being.

In the opinion of this author, *no* complementary therapy treatment whatsoever should be given to pregnant women who have epilepsy, as even the relaxation factor from simple massage may be sufficient in some to trigger a fit. If a practitioner takes the (unwise) decision to treat epileptic clients (even when not pregnant) they should have the knowledge, skills and relevant equipment to deal with an epileptic fit. Similarly, expectant mothers with cardiac disease should not be treated with reflexology, as pregnancy exerts an abnormal pressure on the heart and cardiovascular system which should be monitored closely, and the impact of reflexology could compromise the mother's condition further.

Mothers with pre-existing diabetes mellitus who require insulin (this may increase during pregnancy) should not be treated with reflexology, but those who have non-insulin-dependent diabetes, including those who develop the temporary diabetes of pregnancy, can be treated gently. They may, however, benefit from the advice to eat a small carbohydrate meal prior to treatment and the therapist should have some dry biscuits available in the consulting room in case the mother reacts to the treatment by becoming hypoglycaemic.

REFLEXOLOGY TREATMENT DURING PREGNANCY

The main emphasis of generic reflexology is on restoring and maintaining homeostasis, aiding relaxation and easing symptoms of stress. In pregnancy, this involves helping women to cope with the psychological and emotional demands, relieving pain and anxiety in labour and postnatally, to aid adaptation to parenthood and the establishment of breastfeeding. Reflex zone therapy goes one step further: specific techniques can be employed to ease physical symptoms and prevent pathological complications (see Tiran 2010). In labour, reflexology alleviates pain, while reflex zone therapy might aid uterine action and limit complications such as retained placenta.

The mother's well-being should be assessed before the first and each subsequent treatment in order to determine whether it is appropriate to perform reflexology. She should be asked about her general well-being since the last appointment, fetal movements, the outcome of any visits with the midwife or doctor and how she feels now. If there is any doubt about her health, treatment should be withheld and the mother's midwife consulted for advice. It is also necessary to be alert to the development of pregnancy complications. For example, headaches in early pregnancy are a normal physiological symptom caused by the increase in blood volume in the cerebral blood vessels, whereas headaches in late pregnancy, especially frontal headaches, may be a symptom of worsening pre-eclampsia, requiring immediate medical attention.

The mother's comfort and safety need to be addressed before and during treatment. She should be invited to empty her bladder prior to settling on the treatment couch, and may need to be offered the opportunity to visit the toilet during the course of a treatment; frequency of micturition is a universal problem during pregnancy due to pressure of the uterus on the bladder. It is essential to position the woman sitting upright or in a semi-recumbent position to enable her to converse if she wishes, but more importantly to prevent the effects of supine hypotension from lying flatter, especially in later pregnancy. This occurs because the weight of the heavy uterus compresses the inferior vena cava returning deoxygenated blood to the heart, leading to maternal dizziness and a temporary reduction in fetal oxygenation. If this occurs during treatment, the mother can be turned onto her left side until she feels better. Care should be taken at the end of the treatment to ensure that the woman does not experience further hypotension from sitting or standing up too quickly, and may require support as she gets up. Many women feel slightly dizzy or faint, particularly after the first treatment, and some will become nauseous while the treatment is ongoing. It is better to discontinue the current treatment if this occurs, to avoid additional reactions. If, in earlier pregnancy, the woman has chosen to lie flatter, it is important, at the end of the treatment, to assist her in rising from the couch by advising her to turn onto her side and then push herself up to a sitting position, wait a few seconds and then stand. This prevents postural hypotension and also avoids the danger of overstretching the pelvic ligaments or causing pain in the sacroiliac joint area, both of which are influenced by the hormones progesterone and relaxin during pregnancy.

Pregnant women often have profound and rapid reactions during treatment, significantly more so than those occurring in non-pregnant clients, which is another justification for positioning the mother so that her responses can be observed. It is essential to keep treatments relatively short – the hands-on component of the treatment should last no longer than 35 minutes, even though the whole appointment may last an hour. If the therapist is using a reflex zone therapy approach it is not always essential to undertake a complete treatment; indeed, some physiological conditions respond with just one or two treatments of no more than 10 minutes' duration, with no further appointments being necessary. These include nausea and vomiting, constipation, carpal tunnel syndrome and heartburn (Tiran 2010). Whilst the treatment will obviously encompass the entire surface of both feet, no specific *stimulation* of any reflex points should be undertaken unless it is clinically relevant.

The uterus, fallopian tube and ovary points, and the points for the pituitary gland, *should not be stimulated at all* in pregnancy, and therapists should merely pass over these reflex points. It is of concern that some schools of reflexology teach students to 'massage' the pituitary gland zone during a normal relaxation treatment but this is completely inappropriate during pregnancy. *Stimulation* could theoretically trigger hormonal release which may result in miscarriage or preterm labour, whilst *sedation* (pausing on the point) could suppress the normal physiological action of the pituitary, with similar effects. Conversely, no reflex points should be omitted, otherwise the treatment will seem incomplete. The relaxation point (previously termed the solar plexus point) MUST be palpated very lightly. It is neither necessary nor appropriate to press the thumbs deeply into the solar plexus points to achieve relaxation, and can cause severe symptoms to occur in some women, including palpitations, nausea or dizziness, the latter possibly having a temporary adverse effect on the fetus.

BOX 9.1 Pregnancy conditions in which reflexology should be used with extreme caution or avoided

- History of repeated spontaneous abortions
- Preterm labour or spontaneous membrane rupture in this or a previous pregnancy
- Previous stillbirth or history of intrauterine growth retardation in this or a previous pregnancy
- Antepartum haemorrhage in this or a previous pregnancy
- Pre-eclampsia, eclampsia or severe pre-existing essential hypertension
- Multiple pregnancy
- Breech presentation, transverse or unstable lie
- Medical conditions exacerbated by pregnancy, e.g. cardiac disease, diabetes

BOX 9.2 Physiological conditions of pregnancy that may respond to reflexology

- Nausea and vomiting
- Headache and migraine
- Backache, sciatica, sacroiliac joint pain
- Symphysis pubis diastasis
- Constipation and diarrhoea
- Haemorrhoids
- Varicose veins
- Heartburn and indigestion
- Ptyalism (excessive salivation)
- Carpal tunnel syndrome
- Retention of urine from retroverted incarcerated gravid uterus
- Stress, anxiety, muscle tension

CASE STUDY 9.2   GINA

Gina had suffered severe hyperemesis in both her previous pregnancies but this time the problem was worse. She vomited up to 10 times daily and had already been admitted to hospital for rehydration seven times by the 16th week of pregnancy. She attended the complementary therapy (CT) midwife clinic, accompanied by her mother, who walked with a stick. Gina had had a history of neck and back pain before pregnancy and was complaining of lower abdominal pain, for which no cause could be found. On examining her feet, the CT midwife immediately noticed a brown pigmented area over the lower aspect of the inner ankle bone on Gina's left foot, an area corresponding to the symphysis pubis. On closer questioning, it transpired that Gina's 'abdominal' pain was in fact suprapubic and, from a midwifery perspective, seemed to be in keeping with symphysis pubis diastasis. Gina also said that she felt tenderness when the midwife palpated the lower edge of the outer ankle bone on the same foot, the area relating to the hip and sacroiliac joint. The CT midwife intuitively asked Gina's mother the reason for her use of a stick and was told that she had been born with no acetabulum, a fact that was only discovered at the age of 31 when a pelvic X-ray was performed. The CT midwife returned to Gina's feet, working on the spine, neck, hip, sacroiliac joint and symphysis pubis zones. Gina could tolerate only a few minutes' work but reported feeling much better, less nauseated and relieved of much of the pain in her lower abdomen.

The following week Gina arrived looking dreadful and said she had been so severely sick that she had been readmitted to hospital 5 days after the reflexology. However, she agreed to further treatment and again left the clinic feeling much more at ease, both physically and psychologically. On the third week Gina required virtually no reflexology – the vomiting had decreased to just a couple of times a day and the perpetual nausea had ceased. Gina was delighted, needed no further treatment and progressed with her pregnancy with no other complications.

Following delivery, Gina underwent investigations and was found to have an acetabular problem similar to that of her mother, for which she was then able to have treatment.

CASE STUDY 9.3   REBECCA

Rebecca came to see the CT midwife at 22 weeks of pregnancy complaining of constipation and said she had not had her bowels open for 3 weeks. Not surprisingly, she felt dreadful, almost toxic. The midwife performed 10 minutes of reflex zone therapy on two occasions and Rebecca reported bowel movements twice weekly. The treatment was continued regularly to maintain peristaltic action and keep Rebecca comfortable throughout the remainder of the pregnancy, sometimes combined with essential oils or homeopathic remedies when reflexology alone was not sufficient.

CASE STUDY 9.4   ALI

Ali was a clinically obese girl who reported to the CT midwife at 28 weeks with incapacitating carpal tunnel syndrome, which severely compromised her daily life. Hers was one of the worst cases of carpal tunnel syndrome seen by the midwife, who needed to see Ali weekly for the duration of her pregnancy just to keep the discomfort within manageable limits. Treatment was combined with essential oils, homeopathy and acupressure and Ali was taught how to perform reflex zone 'first aid' when the problem kept her awake at night. An added advantage of seeing her so regularly was that discussion of various concurrent psychosocial problems could take place and other physiological complaints could be treated early. Ali's carpal tunnel syndrome was so severe that she required surgery after delivery to correct it more permanently.

INDUCTION OF LABOUR

Starting labour artificially should only be undertaken for specific reasons. It is *not* the role of the reflexologist to attempt to induce labour: it is a medical procedure that carries certain risks. There is a current trend for women to ask their reflexologists to induce labour merely because they are impatient to end the pregnancy and to meet their new baby. However, neither the woman nor the therapist may fully understand the reasons why labour has not yet commenced or the potential complications of attempting to start labour artificially. It is *professionally irresponsible* for independent therapists to agree to stimulate uterine contractions unless adequate consultation has taken place between the therapist, the woman and the midwife or obstetrician. Attempting to force the mother's body into labour before it is ready can precipitate a cascade of events which complicate labour and may be detrimental to both maternal and fetal well-being. Reflexologists should encourage mothers to appreciate that normal pregnancy can last from 37 to 43 weeks' gestation. Before 37 weeks, labour is considered preterm (premature), but medical induction for being 'overdue' is not normally contemplated until 42 weeks' gestation. The date the mother is given is only an *estimated* date of delivery and should not be taken as an absolute.

However, there is evidence to suggest that receiving regular relaxation reflexology in the last few weeks of the pregnancy facilitates the mother's body to work efficiently, commencing labour spontaneously (McNeill et al. 2006).

If the pregnancy extends beyond the 40th week of gestation specific techniques can then be used to stimulate uterine contractions, on condition that the reflexologist has liaised with the midwife or doctor. It is important to note here that the reflex points for the uterus should *not* be stimulated – physiologically contractions begin in the fundal (top) area of the uterus but are triggered from the anterior pituitary gland in the brain; therefore, intermittent and controlled stimulation of the pituitary points should be used to initiate labour. Once contractions are established no further pituitary stimulation should be needed unless circumstances change, as this may result in hyertonic uterine action in which excessively strong contractions put undue constriction on the fetus, potentially reducing the oxygen supply and leading to fetal distress.

REFLEXOLOGY DURING LABOUR

Reflexology can be extremely relaxing, pain-relieving and psychologically comforting during labour. However, some women dislike being touched in labour and will not wish to receive reflexology at this time, so the therapist should bear this in mind. Reflexology during labour may occasionally be provided by the midwife caring for the woman as an adjunct to normal care, or the mother may have requested the presence of her reflexologist at the birth. If she is having her baby at home, this is fairly easily arranged, although the midwife still needs to be informed. If the baby is to be born in hospital the therapist will need to make the necessary arrangements early in pregnancy. This includes obtaining permission from the midwifery managers to be present on hospital premises. It is the prerogative of the mother to be accompanied by whomever she wishes when she is in her own home. However, on hospital premises there may be rules regarding the number of people permitted to be with her in the labour room at any one time, so this may need to be discussed in advance with the mother and her intended birthing partner. Normal labour can last any length of time up to 24 hours, so it is essential that the reflexologist attends to his or her own well-being and plans accordingly. Hydration and prevention of hypoglycaemia are important, as is keeping cool (labour wards can be very hot).

Reflexology can aid overall relaxation and relief of stress and anxiety, in which case a general treatment will be administered. The foremost hormonal activity in labour is that of oxytocin, which initiates contractions, but the output of this hormone from the pituitary gland can be suppressed by stress hormones such as cortisol (Field & Diego 2008). Thus, helping the mother to remain calm by providing reflexology as a stress-relieving strategy can indirectly influence the progress and outcome of labour and the birth. Specific areas can be treated for pain relief; simple pressure applied to the heels can be very effective during contractions. Other symptoms such as nausea and feelings of panic can also be treated by the reflexologist but communication with the midwife is essential if the mother's condition deviates from normal; labour is a dynamic event in which the situation can change rapidly.

Many women labour on the floor, standing, sitting, in the 'all fours' position, leaning over a birthing ball or constantly changing position, and it may be necessary to perform reflexology with the woman in whatever position she has adopted for most comfort. It is unlikely that a full treatment will be given during labour and the therapist must adapt in accordance with the woman's preferences, sometimes even refraining from undertaking the treatment. In many respects, the reflexologist provides moral and emotional support and should accept that physical treatment is not always appropriate or desirable. It is also unlikely that treatment will be continued during the second stage of labour (the birth of the baby), but reflexology can be helpful in the third stage (delivery of the placenta and membranes). However, it is not appropriate for an independent therapist to interfere with the progress of placental separation and delivery, unless invited by the midwife to do so and with a good understanding of the physiopathology.

POSTNATAL REFLEXOLOGY

Following delivery, reflexology can be used to treat women with physiological discomforts of the puerperium, including constipation, haemorrhoids, perineal discomfort and inadequate lactation. Relief from ongoing discomfort following epidural anaesthesia, such as backache, neck pain or headache, can also be obtained. It is especially beneficial for mothers with a history of, or predisposition to, postnatal depression, although treatment may need to be continued for some time after the birth. Indeed, the therapist who provides regular treatments and comes to know the mother well is in an invaluable position to recognise changes in her psychological well-being, which may indicate developing postnatal depression, and to encourage her to seek specialist medical help.

CONCLUSION

Reflexology offers a gentle yet powerful tool for assisting women during pregnancy, labour and the postnatal period. It can be performed regularly for general health and well-being, or intermittently for specific disorders and discomforts, as well as for relief of pain, anxiety and other symptoms during labour (Box 9.2). Practitioners who specialise in using reflexology to treat pregnant and childbearing women *must* have a thorough knowledge and understanding of physiological changes and possible complications, as well as an appreciation of the conventional maternity services. Reflexology for this client group is complementary to any orthodox maternity care provided.

REFERENCES

Chuang, C.H., Doyle, P., Wang, J.D., Chang, P.J., Lai, J.N., Chen, P.C., 2006. Herbal medicines used during the first trimester and major congenital malformations: an analysis of data from a pregnancy cohort study. Drug Saf. 29 (6), 537–548.

Dept of Health, 2007. Maternity matters: choice, access and continuity of care in a safe service. Department of Health, London.

Dhany, A., 2008. Essential oils and massage in intrapartum care. Pract. Midwife 11 (5), 34–39.

Ejindu, A., 2007. The effects of foot and facial massage on sleep induction, blood pressure, pulse and respiratory rate: crossover pilot study. Complement. Ther. Clin. Pract. 13 (4), 266–275.

Field, T., Diego, M., 2008. Cortisol: the culprit prenatal stress variable. Int. J. Neurosci. 1, 1181–1205.

Lythgoe, J., Metcalfe, A., 2008. Birth of a midwifery acupuncture service. Pract. Midwife 11 (5), 25–29.

McNeill, J.A., Alderdice, F.A., McMurray, F., 2006. A retrospective cohort study exploring the relationship between antenatal reflexology and intranatal outcomes. Complement. Ther. Clin. Pract. 12 (2), 119–125.

Mitchell, M., Allen, K., 2008. Breech presentation and the use of moxibustion. Pract. Midwife 11 (5), 22–24.

O'Hara, C., 2007. UK voluntary self-regulation by January 2008? Clinical Reflexology News Autumn 23, 3–7.

National Collaborating Centre, 2008. Routine care of the healthy pregnant woman. Clinical guideline March 2008. Last viewed online at www.nice.org.uk/nicemedia/ pdf/CG62FullGuidelineCorrectedJune2008 January 2009.

Tiran, D., 2000. Clinical aromatherapy for pregnancy and childbirth, second ed Edinburgh, Churchill Livingstone.

Tiran, D., 2004. Nausea and vomiting in pregnancy: an integrated approach to care. Elsevier, Edinburgh.

Tiran, D., 2010. Reflexology in pregnancy and childbirth: a definitive text for healthcare professionals. Elsevier, Edinburgh.

Williams, J., Mitchell, M., 2007. Midwifery managers' views about the use of complementary therapies in the maternity services. Complement. Ther. Clin. Pract. 13 (2), 129–135.

FURTHER READING

Tiran, D., 2008. Bailliere's midwives' dictionary. Elsevier, Edinburgh.

Tiran, D., 2010. Reflexology in pregnancy and childbirth: a definitive text for healthcare professionals. Elsevier, Edinburgh.

Tiran, D., 2010. Teach yourself positive pregnancy, second ed. Hodder Headline, London.

USEFUL RESOURCES

www.expectancy.co.uk – Expectant parents' complementary therapies consultancy – provides courses and information for reflexologists, accredited by the University of Greenwich and the Federation of Holistic Therapists, as well as services for mothers, including advice on the safe use of complementary therapies in pregnancy and childbirth, and a 'morning sickness' telephone consultancy.

www.babycentre.co.uk – an excellent website, aimed at parents, but also useful for professionals, on everything related to conception, pregnancy, childbirth, postnatal and baby care.

Teaching parents to use reflexology

10

Liz Tipping, with a contribution from Jenny Gordon

ABSTRACT

This chapter will help reflexologists to teach parents how to employ reflexology and foot massage techniques for their children. The chapter will explore different styles of teaching and learning, and how to ensure that parental learning has taken place. The focus is on teaching parents whose babies or children are ill, although the principles can be also applied to teaching those whose children are fit and healthy. When teaching a baby's parents, the focus is on understanding the baby's non-verbal communication to gain an understanding of when and how a reflexology treatment should be given.

KEY WORDS

Teaching, children, babies, parents, teaching styles, learning environment.

INTRODUCTION

Reflexology can be a valuable aid to the treatment and care of babies and children, both those who are healthy and those who are unwell. Reflexology builds on the concept of touch and massage, which has become extremely popular and

DOI: 10.1016/B978-0-7020-3167-0.00010-X

is well researched in the field of paediatrics (Field 2000). However, the opportunities for qualified practitioners to provide regular reflexology treatments for children may be limited by a variety of factors; for example if the baby is asleep or the parent is attending to other siblings. Significantly, teaching parents to give reflexology treatments to their child will be far more beneficial, helping to strengthen the bond between them and helping the parents to overcome any negative emotions associated with the baby's or child's condition. Additionally, reflexology can give them some manual skills to treat different conditions which may affect their baby or child, such as colic in infants or pain in those who are ill.

When working with babies, it is particularly important that a parent gives the treatment rather than the therapist; the parent will know the baby best and will have more understanding of, and the ability to interpret non-verbal language cues, which will enable him or her to work effectively and safely with the baby. Older children too can benefit from reflexology, but the frequency, style and manner of the treatment needs to incorporate their changing lifestyle. Parents may need to be encouraged to provide reflexology for general relaxation at times which suit the child's lifestyle, such as fitting around homework, extracurricular activities and home life. Reflexology with children and babies should be fun, using nursery rhymes with babies, which they will quickly come to associate with specific movements. Examples include 'Incey Wincey Spider' when working the spine reflex zone, and 'This Little Piggy' when working over the toes. For older children, individualised stories can be used, which can be adapted as the child grows or the reason for the treatment alters. For boys, reflexology may provide relief of fatigue and muscle stiffness after playing sports; for teenage girls it could be incorporated as part of a beauty treatment and include a manicure or hairstyling. Whatever the treatment is called, it could become a very special time between parent and child, offering an opportunity for a child to open up about any worries or concerns.

If the child is ill and the parents have been given a diagnosis of a life-threatening illness, they may have feelings of hopelessness, despair and guilt. They may feel that they could have done more to prevent the situation and this may lead to an element of rejection of the child, a 'pulling back' in an attempt to protect themselves from grief. In this case, the baby may then be denied the positive touch which is fundamental for survival, and teaching reflexology techniques at this time offers the parents a positive role in the care of their baby/child. Within the confines of a hospital, giving touch to fragile babies and children requires sensitivity and mindfulness (see Ch. 5) and the practitioner needs to be sensitive to the emotional well-being of the parents (Tipping 2005). Parents, concerned about the stability of their child's condition, may be fearful and lack confidence to touch and handle them, so need encouragement to touch in a gentle, sympathetic and positive way (Tipping 2002) (see Case Study 10.1).

CASE STUDY 10.1

Michael was born at 34 weeks' gestation with mild respiratory problems requiring oxygen therapy, intravenous fluids and antibiotics. Although this baby was not seriously ill, the intensive care unit environment was enough for the mother to think that her newborn baby may not survive. She was frightened of touching her baby in case she became too emotionally involved, but she was encouraged to use containment holds, and given help to understand her baby's non-verbal language. Later, when Michael's condition was more stable, reflexology techniques were taught to the mother. The mother was so grateful for the opportunity to hold her baby in this way that she later sent a letter of thanks to the staff:

"Thank you so much for helping me to hold my little boy when he really needed it most. I was so scared that if I loved him too much, and then he was taken away, that I would fall apart. Your kind reassurance and support gave me the confidence to believe that he was perhaps going to be all right and that he needed me to be there."

Negative emotions associated with learning can inhibit the parents' ability to retain information or may compromise their manual dexterity (Antonacopoulou & Gabriel 2001). If the baby or child is extremely ill, the parents may have a fear of touching them, which can inhibit their interaction and be devastating for the parents and the child. Rather than seeing himself as a primary caregiver in this situation, the father may view his role as one of support for the mother and other children (Deeney et al. 2009), which may be due to a feeling of lack of control (Arockiasamy et al. 2008). Teaching a father how to use reflexology techniques can be empowering, helping him to regain a sense of purpose in the care of his infant. In the event of life-threatening or terminal illness, parents are totally unprepared on all levels to deal with the situation (Milstein & Raingruber 2007) and it is on these occasions that healing measures such as reflexology become of paramount importance.

INDICATIONS FOR TREATING BABIES WITH REFLEXOLOGY

There are many benefits which come from teaching parents to use reflexology techniques with their baby or small child. It can help the parents to regain an element of control at a time when they are feeling uncertain and insecure, especially if the baby has been admitted to a potentially intimidating environment, such as a neonatal unit or ward (Figs 10.1, 10.2). Importantly, reflexology can induce a relaxation response in the giver as well as the recipient. To aid relaxation of the parent it may be appropriate to offer them a treatment, so any anxiety that they have is diminished and not passed to the baby. This will also facilitate the release of prolactin in mothers to aid lactation, and may reduce the impact of postnatal depression and anxiety, through the release of oxytocin (Tipping & Mackereth 2000). If this treatment is carried out with the parent holding the baby, both should benefit from the treatment.

Reflexology techniques can also be taught to parents to enable them to treat their baby or child when it is suffering from symptoms such as colic. This condition, whilst being very common, can be upsetting for the parents because they see the baby in distress, crying for long periods of time, leaving them stressed, helpless and deprived of sleep. Benedbaek et al. (2001) showed a significant improvement in symptoms of colic in a group of babies (n = 63) who received reflexology when compared to the control group.

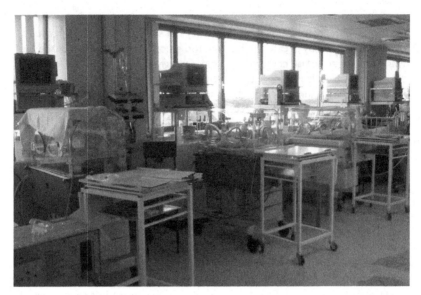

FIG. 10.1 General view of a neonatal unit.

The author suggests that a treatment should be given about 1 hour before the usual onset of symptoms as suggested for massage by Carpenter & Epple (2009), thus helping to calm the baby and the parents, and limiting the severity of the impending colic, or possibly even preventing it from occurring. Other symptoms common in children have also been shown to respond to reflexology, including constipation (Bishop et al. 2003) and reduction of pain (Stephenson 2000, 2003; Lacey 2002), and offering a positive intervention for parents to use when their baby is troubled by problems such as teething, earache or tonsillitis.

Field et al. (2001) argue that touch deprivation can lead to suppression of the immune system, leading to a higher incidence of infections, and it has been suggested that reflexology may strengthen the immune system, although much of this work has been done with adults (see Ch. 2). Providing regular touch therapies, such as reflexology helps to promote positive and health-enhancing contact between parent and child.

Teaching parents to become involved in the child's care also has the potential to minimise the 'medicalisation' of the child's condition (Illich 1979), which occurs in hospital when the child is treated by an 'expert'. This is especially significant in long-term conditions, which can take many months to resolve, or where a life-limiting illness is present. Where appropriate, teaching parents reflexology techniques enables them to use the intervention at home; this helps to support the overall management and care of the child with ongoing medical conditions. A family-centred approach where the parents are actively involved in their child's treatment may help families to feel that they are integral to the treatment. Parents often feel helpless and disempowered during their child's treatment, and involving them in a proactive way may contribute to improving treatment outcomes and the child's well-being. Field and colleagues have completed a number of research studies teaching parents to massage their children, with evidence of improvement in a variety of outcomes (Field et al. 1997, 2000, 2001).

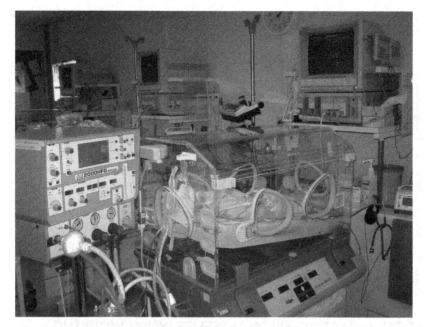

FIG. 10.2 A neonatal incubator: perhaps a parent's first view of their child.

CONTRAINDICATIONS AND PRECAUTIONS

The baby must be assessed on an individual basis prior to each treatment/ teaching session, observing non-verbal cues and taking into account the current condition. Newborn babies can easily become overstimulated by reflexology, as their experience of sights and sounds is intense during the first few weeks of life (Carpenter & Epple 2009). The Meissner corpuscles (the main touch receptors in the skin) are very tightly packed together at birth, so babies may experience a reflexology treatment more intensely than adults, which could be very stimulating or deeply relaxing. Observing cues is essential to determine the optimum duration and frequency of treatment. The skin of a neonate is often fragile, depending on maturity and age, and it may be appropriate to wait until the skin has matured before reflexology is attempted; the skin should be carefully inspected prior to each reflexology treatment. If the baby has an unstable temperature care should be taken to avoid the baby becoming either too hot or too cold during the treatment.

If there is any cerebral irritation, infection, unstable blood pressure, respiratory difficulty, blood glucose fluctuations, congenital heart conditions, abnormal platelets or haematological disorders, the baby should not be treated without the permission of the paediatrician. If the practitioner is in any doubt about the safety and appropriateness of treating a baby on a particular occasion, she or he should discuss this with the relevant health professional, especially if the child is receiving any medications, or their condition has deteriorated.

When a child's condition is very unstable, excessive handling can be overstimulating and reflexology may not be appropriate. However, with skills and sensitivity, a reflexology treatment can be adapted to the needs of a fragile infant, and become a positive and memorable experience for both parent and baby (Case Study 10.2).

CASE STUDY 10.2

Annie had been born very prematurely, at 27 weeks' gestation; by 4 months she had severe brain damage and still required oxygen and ventilation to aid breathing. Although she was often unstable and distressed, she responded well to gentle touch and quiet talk, and appeared to relax when her hands were stroked. As a result, after consultation with the paediatrician, it was decided to teach the parents some simple reflexology techniques. Annie's family were taught how to work up the whole of the feet and hands in circular movements, paying special attention to the solar plexus and lung reflex zones. Her parents were taught containment holds and how to interpret her cues, so if Annie started to become overstimulated, they could revert to this hold to help her settle. The parents found it very helpful to be able to do something positive for their baby at a time when they felt out of control, and Annie benefited from having family around her who could help her to become settled and calm.

LEGAL AND PROFESSIONAL ISSUES WHEN WORKING WITH CHILDREN

If the reflexologist is employed in an environment in which working with children is part of the job description, professional indemnity insurance cover will be provided by the employer. It is mandatory that anyone working with children (and other vulnerable groups) has had a Criminal Records Bureau (CRB) disclosure search performed, a procedure which is normally undertaken by the employer before appointment. It is worth noting that a CRB check undertaken by an employer is *not* transferable and repeat searches may need to be done if the reflexologist changes place of practice.

However, reflexologists working in private practice should ensure they have their own professional indemnity insurance and an up-to-date CRB check, generally required to be updated at least every 3 years. The individual is responsible for ensuring that this has been done, and a fee is payable, which may be anything between £50 and £150, depending on geographical area and the availability of organisations registered to undertake CRB checks. Recommendations for safe practice need to be in place prior to teaching parents. The parent should be observed using the techniques that have been taught, and they should have an understanding of what they are doing and why. It is important that parents know when to stop using reflexology (contraindications) and when to ask for help (Wall 2002).

Practitioners must be able to respond sensitively and appropriately to the needs of children and babies, and should also acknowledge the needs of the parents to care for their own child. It is important that consent is gained from the parent *and* the child before any touch, massage, reflexology or other treatment is given. Older children can be asked directly, although parental consent is also needed, but in the case of babies, it is respectful to obtain implied consent by observing the non-verbal cues (Fig. 10.3). Consent to manual treatments does not necessarily have to be written (i.e. signed) by the parent or child, but in the

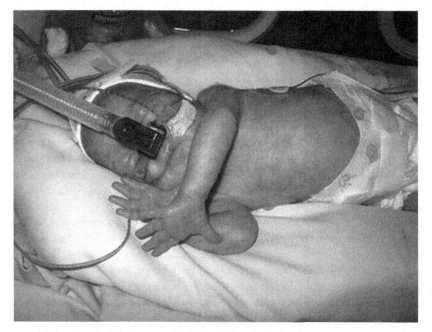

FIG. 10.3 A sick baby demonstrating the ability to say 'no' to touch.

absence of written consent it is usual for the practitioner to record in their notes that consent to treatment was given and how this was achieved. Treatment by a practitioner should always be in the presence of the parent/guardian, after permission has been gained from the baby by observation of cues.

If the reflexologist is working in a hospital setting, protocols and guidelines will need to be written according to individual work environments. These documents are standard in institutional settings and are intended as a means of protecting the client/patient, their relatives and the professionals involved in giving care. Protocols and guidelines do not inform the practitioner precisely what to do in the treatment, but should cover how and where records (notes) are maintained, confidentiality issues, consent and how to deal with issues of concern. If the reflexologist is employed, protocols and guidelines are usually required in order for him or her to take advantage of the institution's vicarious liability insurance cover; conversely, failure to comply with the requirements laid down in the protocols may invalidate the individual practitioner's right to indemnity insurance cover.

TEACHING REFLEXOLOGY TO PARENTS

Teaching parents to provide reflexology for their child requires the reflexologist to adapt his role from one of clinical expert to that of a teacher/facilitator (Mackereth et al. 2006). In doing so, she or he will need to develop new skills in how to teach, and should have an understanding of different learning styles to aid this process (see Box 10.1). For all therapists, continuing education is important to maintain competency in both the therapeutic modality and in teaching. It is important to remember that parents are already under considerable pressure at this time, and are faced with many changes, including the normal disruption which results from the addition of a new baby to the family, or great stress if the child is very ill. It is therefore vital that the reflexologist is sensitive to these pressures and paces the teaching according to the circumstances and learning ability of the individual parent(s), using a range of teaching styles and accepting the need to repeat aspects which may be more difficult for some to grasp. Parents who are interested in using reflexology techniques with their baby may previously have received reflexology treatments themselves, so are likely to have an understanding of the effects of treatment from their own experience. Infant massage is hugely popular amongst new parents and in some cases, if the teacher was also a qualified reflexologist, the parents may have been taught simple reflexology techniques whilst learning infant massage. However, the teaching of reflexology with infant massage is not standard practice in the UK.

When using any touch therapy with a baby the practitioner must have an in-depth knowledge of infant behavioural cues in order to interpret whether the baby is enjoying the experience and to understand when any intervention can start or must stop. Treatment should only be performed when the baby is in a quiet, alert state, rather than drowsy, in a light or deep sleep, or when agitated and crying. Optimally, the baby will be bright and alert, make eye contact, have relaxed, smooth movements and will be the most receptive to any intervention. Reflexology treatments that respect developmental limitations and are responsive to the infant's behavioural cues are likely to be more effective. A self-regulatory balance is the ability to make a smooth transition between states, having levels of awareness between sleeping, waking, active and distressed (Kenner & McGrath 2004). The ability to move between states shows a maturing of neurobehavioural organisation and is therefore a key to the status of the developing brain, which are individual and reflect the infant's ability to adapt to his/her environment.

THE LEARNING ENVIRONMENT

Babies can easily be over stimulated, especially when they are unwell or premature; therefore, the therapeutic environment should be as calm and quiet as possible – even quiet, relaxing music may overstimulate an already overstressed baby. As the baby is likely to be lying supine for a treatment, ceiling lights may be too bright and carefully positioned lamps may be better. Natural light can be acceptable but direct bright sunlight can overstress the baby. Calming techniques such as swaddling may help the baby to stay calm. Teaching the parents to use reflexology techniques will enable the child to be treated little and often without fear of being overstimulated, and only when the baby is seen to consent.

If the reflexologist normally uses a medium such as oils or cream when giving a treatment, consideration should be given to what is suitable for use with babies. It has been established that talcum powder is not recommended for use, especially with children (Silver et al. 1996). As babies will often suck their toes, the medium used must be ingestible. Suitable oils are organic cold-pressed vegetable oil such as sunflower or grapeseed, which are absorbed easily and are not harmful if digested, unlike mineral oils which stay on the surface and may be harmful if ingested. Nut-based oils, such as sweet almond and hazelnut oil are *not* recommended as they could precipitate nut allergy, inducing anaphylactic shock. All oils should be skin tested prior to use on a baby to ensure there is no adverse reaction (Carpenter & Epple 2009). It is important to note that *no* essential oils should be used on or near small or ill babies, either in burners or carrier oils. The baby will inhale the essential oil molecules – and therefore the chemicals in the oils – which may be harmful, may interfere with the immature immunological system and may trigger respiratory problems. The chemicals in the oils are too stimulating for the immature nervous system, and in the longer term, odour association with the reflexology treatment may cause the baby to display negative cues.

LEARNING STYLES

Honey and Mumford (1992) identified four stages in the learning process: activist, reflector, theorist and pragmatist. Activists need to be involved in the experience, whereas reflectors ask questions about the process and observe closely, theorists need structure to the learning process and like handouts, and pragmatists will already have been observing closely and be very attentive but also need structure and clarity (Mackereth & Carter 2006) (Box 10.1). Most adults may be unaware that they have a preferred learning style, highlighting the need for multiple strategies, incorporating visual, kinesthetic and auditory learning styles. It is important to teach the parents the benefits of reflexology through information-giving, facilitating discussion, demonstrating techniques and enabling the parents to observe the effects of treatment (Collins 2004). Recent research by Frankel (2009) showed that adult learners prefer visual or kinesthetic learning, while Beck et al. (2002) suggested that active learning is far more effective than passive learning. Teaching on a one-to-one basis enables the therapist to adjust to the individual needs of the parents, so they can learn at their own pace, thus maintaining confidence in their ability to acquire the skills involved. For those parents who have not had reflexology themselves, enabling them to experience a treatment can be helpful and gives them the opportunity to feel the pressures and techniques used.

When teaching reflexology techniques to parents, it is recommended that the therapist uses an appropriately dressed doll to demonstrate the strokes. The doll should be treated as a baby, offering a role model for the parents, and allowing the therapist to observe the parent–baby interaction so that he or she can guide the parents in a non-judgemental manner (Carpenter & Epple 2009). It also allows the therapist to ensure that the parent has mastered the techniques adequately and can observe and act on the baby's cues effectively. Handouts summarising the reflexology techniques used in the session provide visual guidance, and can be used in the home environment as a prompt for the parent when the therapist is not available.

If the reflexologist is giving the treatment to a baby or child, he should allow sufficient time for the child to get to know him or her before commencing the hands-on component. When demonstrating directly on the baby or observing the parents giving a treatment to their baby, care must be taken if the baby has any intravenous infusions, monitors or other equipment attached to it, to ensure that catheters and wires are not displaced. Ill babies may require frequent blood samples to be taken and other investigations, some of which are painful, and this may lead to the baby becoming ultrasensitive to touch in some areas. As the heels of the feet are often the area of the baby's body from which blood samples are taken, the feet may be very sensitive, potentially making reflexology difficult, at least in the beginning (see Case Study 10.3). It may also be difficult to access the baby's hands as they may have been used for cannulation, but babies also use their hands to self-calm, sucking their fingers or holding onto clothing. It is important to respect the baby and work with it as much as possible.

BOX 10.1 Learning styles

Activists want to get on with the task, without considering what they really want to learn and what they need to know and do in order to learn the skills. When interested, they will join in the learning session enthusiastically, although they may have to be encouraged to reflect on how the quality of what they do can be improved. Activists learn best from active involvement and learn least from handouts, watching, and direct lectures. These learners will want to work alongside the therapists. Therapists may need to 'rein them in' by using breaks to stop and reflect.

Reflectors usually ponder and question rather than jump in to learn new skills. Reflectors can get distracted by detail, and may think of many different ways of doing the massage, rather than the end point, i.e. giving the massage. They will want to observe repeatedly, and have time to digest what they have seen. They like hearing about the research and the massage experiences of other carers and the patient. In practice, this may mean they will be cautious and need space to work out how and when they want to learn.

Theorists gather information before they attempt a task and like very structured and directed ways of working. They learn best from activities which follow a logical sequence, including lectures and demonstrations. Theorists learn least from unstructured, spur of the moment activities, without the aim being clearly articulated. They are not usually comfortable in a group situation, where expressing feelings or other unanticipated contributions may be invited. Well-presented handouts, which include theoretical information are welcomed and reduce wariness associated with trying something new.

Pragmatists like to set clear goals, which is easy to do so long as they can recognise a practical application. They may be intolerant of the theoretical aspects of a situation and are usually focused and keen to achieve their goals. They like to pay attention to detail and have good organisational skills. They may need support in situations where there is no right answer. Pragmatists like to be involved in practical activities and learn least from theoretical lectures and unstructured activities with no clear purpose (Mackereth & Carter 2006, p.103).

ISSUES FOLLOWING DISCHARGE FROM HOSPITAL

It can be a difficult transition for the parents when taking their baby home, especially if she or he remains on oxygen therapy or requires continuing treatment. Whilst in hospital a health professional is always available, but once home the parents must cope alone, which can reduce their confidence and leave them feeling isolated. Parents may also have difficulties when the home has been converted to accommodate medical equipment, or the continued presence of medical personnel may become an intrusion (Kirk et al. 2005). The parents may have lost contact with friends and neighbours if the period of hospitalisation has been prolonged, and teaching reflexology techniques at this time will help them to regain confidence in handling and bonding with the baby.

CASE STUDY 10.3

James was born spontaneously at 26 weeks' gestation, and weighed only 980 g and required ventilation for 3 months. He had had emergency surgery twice, numerous infections requiring antibiotics, prolonged jaundice, prolonged oxygen therapy for chronic lung disease and a delay in tolerating full milk feeds. James still continued to posit and suffered from colic on discharge from hospital, so his parents were taught reflexology and massage to help with this. Due to the daily blood sampling from his heels whilst in hospital, his feet were very sensitive and he pulled his feet away when touched and started crying. The therapist encouraged his mother to play with James's feet when he was quietly alert, initially using her tongue but gradually introducing touch with her thumbs, gently encouraging him to learn that not all touch was painful. His reaction slowly improved with each visit, until eventually he could tolerate reflexology and massage on his feet.

RESEARCH ON TEACHING REFLEXOLOGY TECHNIQUES TO PARENTS

Gordon's (2007) randomised, controlled trial taught reflexology to parents for the management of idiopathic (unexplained) constipation in children aged 1–12 years, and aimed to compare the ways in which children responded either to reflexology or to relaxing foot massage performed by their parents and used at home as part of daily care. An earlier study (Gordon 2003) concluded that children and parents respond well to reflexology because it is non-invasive compared to conventional medical treatments. Parents were taught by an experienced nurse-reflexologist in the constipation clinic. They were given written notes and pictures of the techniques to take home to support the practical sessions. Relaxing foot massage was identified as the most appropriate placebo to enable a comparison to be made between the reflexology and the control groups. The study found that reflexology significantly improved the condition compared to massage and control. All studies have limitations and this one was no exception; however, the study has demonstrated that reflexology has a role in improving outcomes for children when taught to parents and used as an adjunct to standard treatment of idiopathic constipation. Small studies have been undertaken to investigate the effect of teaching parents to use massage for their children (Barlow et al. 2008), on teaching partners to give reflexology to adults with cancer

(Stephenson et al. 2007) and on teaching women with depression or pre-menstrual disorder to self-administer reflexology (Kim et al. 2004; Lee 2006). However, this is the only randomised, controlled study to date in which reflexology is practiced by parents in a paediatric setting, and further well-designed studies are needed.

CONCLUSION

It is possible, and even desirable, to involve parents in the treatment of their baby/child by teaching them to perform simple reflexology treatments. It is important to acknowledge that the distress experienced in a hospital environment can stay with the parent(s) for many years to come, undermining confidence and child-rearing skills. Teaching reflexology techniques and helping the parents to develop an understanding of their baby's body language can empower parents and give them a positive role to play with the care of their baby. When taught these techniques, parents learn to understand their babies, often better than the nursing staff.

The impact of touch alone and the psychosocial effects on the whole family from the close relationship which forms during and after this type of treatment is invaluable and contributes greatly to the overall well-being of the child and the parents. Due to the paucity of good-quality research evidence it is not currently possible to recommend the best techniques to be used. It is suggested that reflexologists assess their paediatric clients to determine the aims of any treatment, then consider whether teaching a particular technique to the parents will assist in achieving those goals. Parents, carers and older children should be involved in any discussions, planning and evaluation of this type of treatment. A simplified form of reflexology which can be given by the parents can be taught fairly easily and provides more benefits than problems.

REFERENCES

Antonacopoulou, E., Gabriel, Y., 2001. Emotion, learning and organisational change: towards an integration of psychoanalytic and other perspectives. J. Organisational Change 14 (5), 435–451.

Arockiasamy, V., Holsti, L., Albersheim, S., 2008. Father's experiences in the neonatal intensive care unit: a search for control. Paediatrics 121 (2), e215–e222.

Barlow, J.H., Powell, L.A., Gilchrist, M., Fotiadou, M., 2008. The effectiveness of the Training and Support Program for parents of children with disabilities: a randomized controlled trial. J. Psychosom. Res. 64 (1), 55–62.

Beck, A., Bennett, P., Wall, P., 2002. Communication studies: the essential introduction. Routledge, London.

Benedbaek, O., Viktor, J., Carlsen, K.S., Roed, H., Vinding, H., Christensen, S., 2001. Infants with colic. A heterogeneous group possible to cure? Treatment by pediatric consultation followed by a study of the effect of zone therapy on incurable colic. Ugeskr. Laeger 163 (27), 3773–3778.

Bishop, E., McKinnon, E., Weir, E., Brown, D.W., 2003. Reflexology in the management of encopresis and chronic constipation. Paediatr. Nurs. 15 (3), 20–21.

Carpenter, P., Epple, A., 2009. Infant massage: the definitive guide for teaching parents. Ditto International, Buckinghamshire.

Collins, J., 2004. Education techniques for lifelong learning: principles of adult learning. Radiographics 24 (5), 1483–1489.

Deeney, K., Lohan, M., Parkes, J., Spence, D., 2009. Experiences of fathers of babies in intensive care. Paediatr. Nurs. 21 (1), 45–47.

Field, T., 2000. Touch therapy. Churchill Livingstone, London.

Field, T., Hernandez-Reif, M., Seligman, S., Krasnegor, J., Sunshine, W., 1997. Juvenile rheumatoid arthritis: benefits from massage therapy. J. Pediatr. Psychol. 22 (5), 607–617.

Field, T., Cullen, C., Diego, M., Hernandez-Reif, M., Sprinz, P., Beebe, K., et al., 2001. Leukemia immune changes following massage therapy. J. Bodywork Movement Ther. 3, 1–5.

Frankel, A., 2009. Nurses' learning styles: promoting better integration of theory into practice. Nurs. Times 105 (2), 24–27.

Gordon, J., 2003. Reflexology pilot study report. The Royal Hospital for Sick Children, Edinburgh.

Gordon, J.S., 2007. The effectiveness of reflexology as an adjunct to standard treatment in childhood idiopathic constipation: a single blind randomised controlled trial. Napier University, Edinburgh.

Honey, P., Mumford, A., 1992. The manual of learning styles. Peter Honey, Maidenhead.

Illich, I., 1979. Limits to medicine. Marion Boyars, London.

Kenner, C., McGrath, J.M. (Eds.), 2004. Developmental care of newborns & infants: a guide for health professionals. Mosby, Philadelphia.

Kim, Y.S., Kim, M.Z., Jeong, I.S., 2004. The effect of self-foot reflexology on the relief of premenstrual syndrome and dysmenorrhea in high school girls. Taehan Kanho Hakhoe Chi 34 (5), 801–808.

Kirk, S., Glendinning, C., Callery, P., 2005. Parent or nurse? The experience of being a parent of a technology-dependent child. J. Adv. Nurs. 51 (5), 456–464.

Lacey, M.D., 2002. The effects of foot massage and reflexology on decreasing anxiety, pain, and nausea in patients with cancer. From Research to Clinical Practice 6 (3), 183–184.

Lee, Y.M., 2006. Effect of self-foot reflexology massage on depression, stress responses and immune functions of middle aged women. Taehan Kanho Hakhoe Chi 36 (1), 179–188.

Mackereth, P.A., Carter, A., 2006. Massage and bodywork: adapting therapies for cancer care. Churchill Livingstone, London.

Mackereth, P.A., Stringer, J., Gray, D., 2006. Therapist as teacher. In: Mackereth, P., Carter, A. (Eds.), Massage & bodywork: adapting therapies for cancer care. Elsevier, Churchill Livingstone.

Milstein, J.M., Raingruber, B., 2007. Choreographing the end of life of a neonate. Am. J. Hosp. Palliat. Med. 24 (5), 343–349.

Silver, P., Sagey, M., Rubin, L., 1996. Respiratory failure from corn starch inhalation: a hazard of diaper changing. Paediatr. Emerg. Care 12 (2), 108–110.

Stephenson, L.N., 2003. Using reflexology for pain management: a review. J. Holist. Nurs. 21 (2), 179–191.

Stephenson, L.N., Weinrich, S.P., Tavakoli, A.S., 2000. The effects of foot reflexology on anxiety and pain in patients with breast and lung cancer. Oncol. Nurs. Forum 27 (1), 67–72.

Stephenson, L.N., Swanson, C.S., Dalton, J., Keefe, F.J., Engelke, M., 2007. Partner-delivered reflexology: Effects on cancer pain and anxiety. Oncol. Nurs. Forum 34 (1), 127–132.

Tipping, E., 2002. Practising in the neonatal area. In: Mackereth, P.A., Tiran, D. (Eds.), Clinical reflexology: a guide for health professionals. Churchill Livingstone, London.

Tipping, E., Mackereth, P.A., 2000. A concept analysis: the effect of reflexology on homeostasis to establish and maintain lactation. Complement. Ther. Nurs. Midwifery 6 (4), 189–198.

Tipping, E., 2005. Adapting touch techniques for the neonate. Connections Spring 1 (9), 6–8.

Wall, A., 2002. Agreeing a standard for infant massage: not a soft touch. J. Neonatal Nursing 8 (3), 93–96.

Teaching parents to use reflexology

Adapted Reflextherapy for pain – an alternative physiotherapy approach

Gunnel Berry

11

ABSTRACT

Evidence for the efficacy of commonly used reflexology techniques in the treatment of patients with low back pain is limited. This chapter describes a method of reflex therapy known as Adapted Reflextherapy, which has been used by the author in NHS and private clinics since 1999, in combination with physiotherapy treatment for pain, including whiplash-associated disorder. Particular emphasis is put on the neurophysiological aspects of pain and speculation of its activity in Adapted Reflextherapy. A series of case studies are presented at the end of the chapter to illustrate this work (Case studies 11.1 to 11.4).

KEY WORDS

Chronic pain, whiplash injury, hypersensitivity, cortical re-organisation, autonomic nervous system, tactile stimulus, adapted reflextherapy, clinical reasoning.

DOI: 10.1016/B978-0-7020-0.00011-1

INTRODUCTION

The author is a physiotherapy clinical specialist in the treatment of chronic and acute pain, who was offered an opportunity, in 1999, to participate in a pilot study of physiotherapy for patients with whiplash injury in a general medical practice (Tobin 2000). Having also studied and practiced generic reflexology for many years, a coincidental event occurred at this time, in which she observed a demonstration of reflexology, using only a single point of application on the feet to achieve a change in symptoms. This caused her to question and challenge her reflexology practice and to consider new ways of working, which resulted in the development of a new style of treatment with its own techniques, working hypotheses and applied clinical reasoning.

Pain, especially chronic pain, is a common reason for physiotherapy referral. Chronic pain affects 15–20% of the population in the United States (Stephenson & Dalton 2003) and one in five adults in Europe (Breivik et al. 2005). It is reported that 20% of all whiplash-injured patients still suffer painful states 6 months after the injury occurred (Malanga & Nadler 2002; Chien & Sterling 2005), and to date there is no known therapy which has proved reliably effective for improving symptoms of patients suffering from chronic disability.

DEFINITION OF ADAPTED REFLEXTHERAPY

Many physiotherapists use reflexology or reflex zone therapy; the term 'reflextherapy' was adopted in 1992 by the Association of Chartered Physiotherapists in Reflextherapy (ACPIRT). This reflects the therapeutic intention of the therapy within physiotherapy practice, as well as embracing the variety of reflexology approaches available. Adapted Reflextherapy (AdRx) is a task-specific, manual, topical, stimulation of short duration to the feet according to the principles of reflexology but with reasoned aspects of neurogenic adaptation in painful states (Berry 2007a). AdRx is practiced according to established standards for physiotherapy practice (Core Standards 2005), including patient consent, assessment and treatment cycle and documentation of outcomes. AdRx has been used to treat patients of all age groups with acute and chronic pain states and has proved particularly effective in reducing hypersensitivity in whiplash-injured patients. Over 200 professionals have been trained to use AdRx in their own work, indicating its transferability across other disciplines.

AdRx uses the original theory of reflexology as a basis to identify areas on the feet which correspond to other parts of the body. However, while reflexology treatment encompasses the whole foot and is intended to be a general health stabilisation technique, AdRx is very specific and seeks out those areas which are specifically relevant to the patient's presentation. Since many physiotherapy patients have musculoskeletal problems, frequently with spinal involvement, and some neurological compromise, AdRx is performed primarily on the reflex zones for the spine. In accordance with most reflexology charts, the area of the spine is represented on the medial longitudinal arches of the feet beginning at the calcaneum representing the sacrum and coccyx, the navicular and cuboid bone representing the lumbar spine and the first metatarsal bone representing the thoracic spine. The cervical spine is represented on the proximal phalanx of the big toe with the right foot representing the right half of the spine and the left foot representing the left half. Foot examination and treatment is convenient and provides a quick overview of the whole spine; frequently, areas of stiffness or tenderness are found in the foot, which, from reflextherapy theory, indicate compromise of spinal structures.

INDICATIONS

Adapted Reflextherapy is used in physiotherapy practice to assess and treat patients of any age who are suffering from some form of pain or discomfort, especially those suffering whiplash-associated disorder (WAD). A whiplash injury is 'an acceleration and deceleration mechanism of energy transfer to the neck' (Hartling et al. 2001), most frequently caused by a road traffic accident, although similar trauma may occur in any situation where the head and neck are exposed to sudden acceleration–deceleration motions (Barnsley et al. 2002). The sudden, rapid change of direction in the movement of the head and neck results in hyperflexion and hyperextension. Fifty per cent of patients with whiplash injury recover within 3 months without the need for medical treatment (Malanga & Nadler 2002); 27% recover in 6 months, but 19–23% are still suffering symptoms after 1 year (Chien & Sterling 2005). There appear to be some adapted central nervous system processing mechanisms at work which assist recovery (Chien et al. 2008), but there is currently no guaranteed effective treatment for those with long-term problems (Atherton et al. 2006). AdRx may be used as the only method of treatment or, more often, in conjunction with other modalities. Most patients referred for treatment of WAD attend between four and six sessions.

CONTRAINDICATIONS AND PRECAUTIONS

Adapted Reflextherapy is undertaken only after a careful assessment of the patient's previous medical history and assessment of the physical and psychological aspects of the pain. There are few contraindications to the use of AdRx: the ACPIRT advises that patients in whom AdRx is inappropriate include those with malignant melanoma; deep vein thrombosis, phlebitis, venous and/or lymphatic inflammation; transplants of heart, kidney or other organs; acute infectious diseases; at risk of ectopic pregnancy; syncope after commencing treatment; known epilepsy; any other concerns regarding medical or behavioural symptoms.

As with conventional reflexology, strict precautions should be applied to patients with neurological disturbance, acute metabolic diseases, first-trimester pregnancy, AIDS and immunosuppressive conditions, psychotic disturbance and schizophrenia, contagious diseases, peripheral vascular disease, tuberculosis or suspected symptoms and diabetes mellitus. Medication may inhibit adverse reactions to therapy; therefore, caution should be exercised in patients who are persistent drug abusers or who are taking prescribed medications, particularly slow-release or long-term medication, e.g. hormone replacement therapy, thyroxine, insulin and antihypertensives.

Adapted Reflextherapy for pain – an alternative physiotherapy approach

HISTORY TAKING AND ASSESSMENT

Adapted Reflextherapy is only applied following a full physiotherapy assessment conducted by a qualified physiotherapist trained in this particular technique. AdRx assessment is incorporated into this process, including a full history of any past road traffic accidents, falls and mishaps, even those which occurred a long time ago and have been almost forgotten. Even minor incidents may have an effect on the neural system, causing neural adaptation (Greening 2006) whilst peripheral inputs will alter the nociceptive afferent barrage proposing an ongoing alteration of the central processing effect (Gracely et al. 1992; Coderre et al. 1993). Sympathetic nervous pathways appear to have a role to play in maintained pain patterns, yet, can also be independent of that pathway, but either may have an accumulative effect (Coderre et al. 1993; Butler et al. 2003) due to a new gene expression, which may be just the 'tip of the iceberg' in the present pain presentation. The assessment process also includes any history of major operations and possible scar formation of fascial structures, dental changes, jaw reconstructions however seemingly insignificant at the time, but which may have a role to play in the current pain presentation. Clinical observations suggest that, in the main, most episodes of unknown pain patterns have an origin of compromise in the neuromusculoskeletal chain, possibly dating back beyond the present clinical presentation and beyond the patient's own recall of such events, although these assumptions are difficult to prove.

Research has shown that the impact of trauma on the body may develop into post-traumatic stress disorder (PTSD) (Rothschild 2000). PTSD includes chronic hyperarousal of the autonomic nervous system (ANS) in addition to 'flashbacks' and avoiding reminders of the trauma. Patients seen in everyday physiotherapy departments may not be diagnosed with PTSD but they may nevertheless have a very minor tendency towards the same neurological pattern of events, which may influence existing pain patterns. The basis of this theory is that increased pain-producing peptide levels are found distally from the primary source of injury in vitro (Eliav et al. 1999) and in vivo after trauma (Guez et al. 2003).

Following the history taking, a physical examination of the whole spine and lower limbs is undertaken, even if the WAD symptoms are located in the shoulder and neck region. Other issues, such as posture compromise (e.g. scoliotic changes), muscle bulk imbalances, leg length difference, circulatory insufficiencies, outcomes of other treatments, shingles and invasion of foreign bodies (tics, wasp stings) can easily be identified and may be relevant to AdRx treatment. This is followed by examination of the feet to elicit further information related to possible areas of compromise in the body. Findings from the physical examination are discussed with the patient. If the patient agrees, the treatment can commence.

TREATMENT APPLICATION OF ADAPTED REFLEXTHERAPY

Adapted Reflextherapy treatment is applied as pressure to the feet, or hands if appropriate, using five handhold techniques. The five handhold techniques are: 'walking', with intermittent pressure and release, to identify stiff segments;

three-point AdRx, using three points of contact on the medial arches of the foot as part of the treatment procedure; spine zone twisting, to aid assessment and treatment; linking, in which pressure is simultaneously applied to two or more points on the feet, similar to the linking used in precision reflexology (Williamson 1999); and a technique called 'thru/thru', another form of partial linking, which has been seen to ease thoracic spine stiffness and involvements of the ribs and myogenic structures associated with the ribs and intercostal nerve impingement.

Interpretation and identification of the feet structures are compared with the patient's clinical presentation and whether it has any clinical relevance. Tactile pressure on sensitive areas on the feet produces pain, which affirms the afferent connection to higher centres. Sporadically, the patient reports sensory changes during treatment episodes such as 'warmth', 'tingling', 'pain running up my leg', 'a funny sensation in the leg' (formication), 'prickling in the back' and lightheadedness. This is a further confirmation of neural involvement suggesting an autonomic nervous system reaction. Whether this is an increase of the sympathetic component of the ANS is speculative. See Sterling and Kenardy (2006) for a discussion of the relationship between post-traumatic stress reaction (PTSR) and sympathetic nervous system changes in whiplash injury. The outcome of the treatment frequently results in an increased (cervical) range of spinal movement and peripheral joint movement in correlation to which area has just been treated. Increased straight leg raising mobility is also frequently noted.

Patients suffering from WAD who do not recover from their symptoms often present with central hypersensitivity tissues (Curatolo et al. 2001) and show widespread mechanical hyperalgesia (Scott et al. 2005), independent of any anxiety, which may indicate poor prognosis (Sterling & Jull 2003). Hypersensitivity is a neurological phenomenon indicating abnormal responses to a normal stimulus that would not usually evoke a response. Some trauma may create hyperalgesia after minor nerve injury with no obvious signs of nerve damage (Greening 2001). The nervi neuorum can become spontaneously active and mechanically sensitive after injury (Greening 2006), and the axonal flow may contain traces of inflammatory cells (Eliav et al. 1999) indicating peripheral involvement in damaged nerve tissue and immunological changes (Marchand et al. 2005). Multiple body systems are activated to respond to the 'fight or flight' situation triggered by injury and pain, including the autonomic nervous and endocrine systems (Van Griensven 2005), and there is an increased probability of immune-cell signalling after peripheral nerve injury which feeds abnormal nociceptive inputs into the dorsal root ganglion (Saab & Hains 2008). Melzack and Wall (1991) introduced the concept of 'plasticity' of the nervous system and suggested that the inter-related activity demand and reaction in the nervous system as a whole reacts, protects and repairs itself in adverse conditions. In AdRx, pressure on the skin is adjusted according to irritability of the tissues. High irritability tissue symptoms require light touch of short duration, which is frequently used in acute inflammatory conditions directly after trauma. Low irritability, as seen in more chronic conditions, necessitates deeper pressure of longer duration being applied to the skin. AdRx treatment is performed with the patient supine to enable the practitioner to assess straight leg raise testing as treatment progresses.

Adapted Reflextherapy for pain – an alternative physiotherapy approach

The early findings of Ingham in 1938 (Ingham 2005) of a correlation between sensory endings on the feet and the soma are supported in contemporary clinical practice by reflexology and reflextherapy practitioners (Quinn et al. 2008), and AdRx has been well justified by conscientious documentation of patient responses and the effectiveness of treatment (Berry 1999, 2003, 2007). Although the inter-relational interpretation and mechanism of action is inconclusive (Tiran & Chummun 2005) this should not exclude the possibility of verification at a later stage. Whilst speculation over the mechanism of action continues, clinical demand for action to improve patients' painful conditions is unrelenting. The ultimate challenge in clinical practice is how to impart a coding system into the physical body which can break the reactive hardware system which has reacted quite naturally to a 'fight and flight' situation.

AdRx may produce counter-irritability whereby the CNS, including the autonomic nervous system, has to react to peripheral tactile sensory stimulus. During AdRx the quantity and quality of neurotransmitters within the neural axonal content change, a phenomenon which has been shown during stroking applications in general massage (Lund et al. 2005) although the mechanism for this is purely speculative. Clinical observations suggest that AdRx facilitates a diagnostic element in addition to effects of the treatment itself, although assessment and identification of tender areas on the feet is undertaken as part of the total physical assessment of the patient. Importantly, physical findings are compared and reasoned before treatment commences.

Trauma involves autonomic responses as well as major musculoskeletal adaptations irrespective of the magnitude. At a molecular level, peptide levels alternate due to inflammatory responses (Greening 2001; Saab & Hains 2008), which can be measured at the primary source of pain as well as at the secondary, distal source. Patients may present with a distal symptom mirroring an injury but on further investigation it is found to be a secondary hyperalgesia (Saab & Hains 2008). The autonomic loop is known to influence ascending primary pathway afferents in the dorsal horn, and the sympathetic portion of the autonomic nervous system may play a role in influencing chronic pain states (Passatore & Roatta 2006).

ADVANTAGES OF ADAPTED REFLEXTHERAPY

Patients report feeling very relaxed during and after treatment, and of being less stressed and anxious, in common with generic reflexology (McVicar et al. 2007; Mackereth et al. 2008). Patients with high irritability of symptoms or poor experience of previous treatments are often fearful of the treatment itself but find AdRx less stressful and less painful than when physiotherapy treatment is given directly on the sensitive tissues. Pain can be relieved and movement function restored in few treatment sessions in a high proportion of patients. The majority of patients make a highly satisfactory recovery and the treatment appears to have predictable results, according to one clinical audit (Berry 2007a). The treatment and its underpinning theory appear to be accurate, in that sensitive areas on the feet correspond closely to the patient's complaint.

DISADVANTAGES OF ADAPTED REFLEXTHERAPY

It has been noted that pain and other associated symptoms may increase within the 24–48 hours after the treatment and are usually worst after the first session (healing crisis). In most cases these effects are mild, but in a few patients are considerable, although not harmful; they are usually temporary and settle down to below the original pain level. It may be considered an unethical disadvantage that pain increases post-treatment, although some patients consider it to be proof of efficacy of treatment.

After treatment, the patient may feel dizzy or lightheaded for an hour or so. They often report feeling tired for up to 24 hours after treatment, enforcing a period of rest and relaxation which, for some, is a novel sensation after suffering continued pain. Some patients find that their protective responses to avoid emotional eruptions are eroded. This may be an unwanted reaction, but conversely some patients are relieved to be able to 'let go' of the emotions related to their pain, which may be associated with stimulation of cognitive stressors finding a mechanism for expression (Watson 1999). Some patients are sceptical about AdRx but most are amazed and relieved that this particular treatment is available, especially in the NHS.

OUTCOME MEASURES

Adapted Reflextherapy uses outcome measures such as a visual analogue scale (VAS) (Kahl & Cleland 2005) to assess pain and MYMOP (Paterson 1996) and percentage of improvements to assess functional and general effects. The prediction of outcome made in AdRx relies on a normally healthy nervous system undergoing a temporary change, albeit long-term in some cases, disrupted by external forces. Less prediction of outcome can be made in conditions where the nervous system is undergoing permanent neuropathological changes such as in multiple sclerosis, Parkinson's disease, motor neurone disease and cerebellar ataxia, due to the lack of full understanding of the aetiology and the synaptic activity and neural adaptations.

THE EVIDENCE BASE

The existence and accuracy of a sensory homunculus on the feet remains to be confirmed. Attempts have been made to measure these distinct areas using action potentials (Pauly 2009) but verification of the documentation remains wanting. Nevertheless, by using the identified areas of sensitivity for application of AdRx on the feet, patients frequently report sensory changes in the specific body area being treated. In addition, they may experience sensory activities in other areas during and/or after the treatment.

It is recognised that the management of chronic pain is multifactorial (Erdmann & Munglani 2000) possibly requiring combined treatment methods addressing both the biological and psychosocial aspects of recovery (Sterling et al. 2005). The concept of 'psychoneuroimmunology' has crept into academic discussions as a means of explaining the complexity of inter-correlations between anatomical systems in relation to chronic pain issues (Alford 2006).

Adapted Reflextherapy for pain – an alternative physiotherapy approach

Generic reflexology has been shown to reduce pain in a variety of clinical groups. Khan et al. (2006) reported reduced foot pain in a female patient, suffering from rheumatoid arthritis, lasting 2–3 days after reflexology although the pain had returned by the time the patient returned for further treatment. Stephenson and Dalton (2003) found temporary reduction of pain in breast cancer patients after reflexology treatment. Tolerance to pain before and after receiving reflexology was shown to be significant compared to sham TENS by Samuel et al. (2003) in their interim findings. Quinn et al. (2008) suggest further work in the treatment of lower back pain using reflexology.

There are no randomised, controlled trials to prove beyond doubt the effects of AdRx. Observational interpretations of AdRx treatments on three patients suffering from chronic spinal pain after injury appear to demonstrate reduced pain, improved mobility and the capability to return to work (Berry 1999). A retrospective analysis of three adolescents suffering from pain and movement dysfunction showed the benefits of AdRx (Berry 2003). Other documentation includes a series of case studies predicting the outcomes of AdRx on patients with WAD (Berry 2007b).

CONCLUSION

Adapted Reflextherapy was developed in 1999 and has since been used as an examination tool and treatment modality, in conjunction with physiotherapy, for acute and chronic spinal pain including cases of whiplash-associated disorder. Although speculation of the origin and pathophysiological mechanism prevails, the outcomes are too persuasive to be ignored. It is recommended that randomised, controlled studies are carried out to confirm the empirical evidence. In the absence of existing effective therapeutic evidence for patients with chronic WAD persistent pain and dysfunctional symptoms, AdRx seems to offer a predictable initiative. The question is whether we are treating the accumulation of secondary hyperalgesia or an area of primary hyperalgesia. It is postulated by the author that we frequently treat secondary hyperalgesia as primary without revealing the primary source. The quandary is how to measure and confirm this theory. Ultimately, the question should be: how do we communicate with the body to influence it to change?

CASE STUDY 11.1

Robert, a 33-year-old man of normal stature with no other medical issues, was referred for physiotherapy after a rear-end vehicular crash in which he had been the driver. Robert's car had been pushed forward and turned 180 degrees to hit the crash barrier in the middle of the road. He returned to work within 48 hours. Being an electrician, he continued to carry equipment, climb ladders and work in small, restricted areas. Eight months later Robert was still suffering from symptoms arising from the incident. At his first visit for AdRx, his main complaint was left-sided neck pain when reaching with the left arm and turning the head to the left. Other symptoms included slight dizziness which developed 2 months after the accident, lower jaw pain, which subsided after 7 months, and abdominal pain which occurred every morning and was associated with a sensation of bladder retention. On examination, Robert's neck movements were generally 75% of normal movements. Pain was not severe – 0–3/10 – but increased after carrying his electrician's toolkit to 4–5/10. Examination on the feet indicated bilateral compromise at the level of the third cervical vertebra. The reflex zone for the second sacral vertebra was sensitive on the left foot, perhaps indicating bladder irritation in addition to stiffness at the level of the left thoracic 7–11 spinal segments. It has been found that the thoracic spine is compromised on impact from a road traffic accident, possibly due to the restrictive action of the seatbelt on the right shoulder (driver), leaving the left side of the thoracic spine free to rotate excessively with force to the right. The opposite would be the case for the passenger on the front seat. The prognosis was that Robert would make 80–99% improvement over a period of 7 weeks following five treatments. By mutual agreement Robert finished his treatment after 4 weeks, considering himself to be 80–99% improved.

CASE STUDY 11.2

Joan was a fit 72-year-old lady who had been suffering from a two-year history of sharp left-sided groin/hip pain. She had undergone manipulation under anaesthetic (MUA) and had a hydrocortisone injection in the hip joint in order to relieve symptoms, but the pain remained static, prevented her from walking far and kept her awake at night. Joan was referred for physiotherapy and received four sessions of standard treatment but full function was not restored. Examination of the feet revealed sensitivity on the reflex zones for the symphysis pubis, which was interpreted as a compromise relating to stiffness. Reduced mobility in the symphysis pubis inhibits normal flexion and extension and rotational integrity of the hip joint. Adverse joint mechanics may result in overloading or underuse of musculogenic structures around the hip, causing groin pain and bursitis in the greater trochanter, together with radiating lower limb pain. AdRx treatment involves a linking technique between the point of contact for the symphysis pubis and the sacroiliac joint reflex zones including point of contact with the lumbosacral area and the hip reflex zones, all on the same side around the ankle (four points of contact) (Fig. 11.1). This technique was carried out once for approximately 4 minutes' continuous pressure on the same areas and Joan experienced immediate pain relief of the groin and hip. It also resulted in a marked increase in range of movement and passive straight leg raising, with a long-lasting effect. Joan needed only one more treatment of AdRx which included sacroiliac/symphysis pubis linking.

Adapted Reflextherapy for pain – an alternative physiotherapy approach

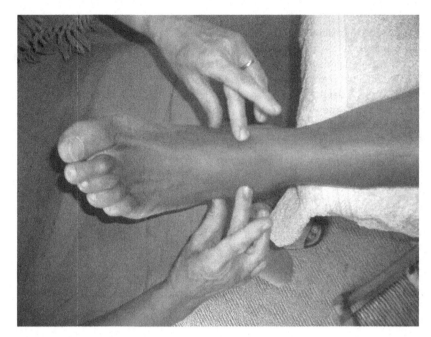

FIG. 11.1 Adapted Reflextherapy using linking technique.

CASE STUDY 11.3

David was a 69-year-old man who had suffered a viral infection of the cerebrospinal fluid 2 years prior to referral for AdRx. He had suffered constant daily headaches ever since, varying in intensity from 2–3/10 to severe pain during a sneezing episode, when the pain rose to 6–7/10.

His medical history revealed a whiplash injury 13 years previously, a minor myocardial infarction 2 years later, a fractured clavicle aged 4, and intermittent pain in the left hip area after a fall in 1968. David had played a lot of rugby and was keen on keeping fit.

On examination, David was clearly in distress with a severe headache and right shoulder stiffness and pain which had not resolved for 2 years. The main aim of his AdRx treatment was to reduce the hyperirritable tissue components. Tactile peripheral input (in the form of massage) appears to offer a mechanism of deregulation in the higher centres and the autonomic nervous system. Guez et al. (2003) found a difference in the peptide content of the cerebrospinal fluid in those patients suffering chronic pain after whiplash injury, as opposed to those who had head and neck pain for other reasons, the increased peptide content being consistent with the chronic pain pattern. Foot examination revealed high irritability on the cerebral areas on the feet (big toes, particularly the plantar aspect). These areas were also red in colour, which was worse on the right than the left foot. Straight leg raising of the left leg produced headaches, whilst tensing of neural tissues when sitting was negative on both legs. There was no indication in the cervical spine reflex zone of neural tension from head movements. There was restricted movement in the right shoulder, with a painful arc between 100 and 140 degrees of flexion, although there was no clear correlation between the headaches and the restricted shoulder joint movement. Symptoms were severe, with moderate irritability of partially neurogenic and arthrogenic origin, but also habituation of pain which can occur after such a long episode of chronic pain (Rothschild 2000). David required long-term AdRx treatment, but after 18 months the headaches had resolved.

CASE STUDY 11.4

Four-year-old Felicity suffered severe dermatitis around all joint folds such as neck, elbows, wrists, hips, knees and ankles and had received 2 years of treatment from a dermatologist. Her itching skin was raw and kept her awake at night due to pain in the joint folds. Other symptoms included lethargy, lack of appetite, constipation, pain on passing urine, lactose intolerance, chronic diarrhoea after mumps, measles and rubella immunisation, pain in the lower back whilst sitting cross-legged in school assembly, and physical activity caused her discomfort in the spine.

On examination of Felicity's feet, a clear rigidity and sensitivity was seen along the whole of the medial arches representing the spinal reflex zones. The reflex zone for the fifth cervical vertebra was particularly tender on both feet, the zone for the junction of the twelfth thoracic and first lumbar vertebrae on both feet was immobile and sensitive and it was thought that Felicity may have sustained a spinal injury from a fall. On questioning her mother, it transpired that Felicity had fallen down the stairs at 18 months old and had also fallen off a slide 3 months prior to attending for AdRx. This leads to an assumption that, as the child grows, neural structures do not adequately accommodate to spinal growth, causing neural compromise and symptoms of adverse neural tension, including abnormal autonomic function. Felicity received seven treatments over a period of 5 months, each session lasting approximately 10 minutes. Areas of most eminent tenderness and stiffness were targeted as they were considered the prime source of her problems. Initially, there was a 24-hour increase in itching symptoms, but there was then a steady improvement in all symptoms as treatment progressed, including less skin irritation and a dramatic change in Felicity's sleeping patterns. School staff noticed a change in her behaviour; she was generally happier, able to join in with other children and was eating better. Two years later, Felicity had a slight recurrence of her condition after falling off a horse but her symptoms settled quickly after two treatments of AdRx.

REFERENCES

Alford, L., 2006. Psychoneuroimmunology for physiotherapists. Physiotherapy 92, 187–191.

Atherton, K., Wiles, N., Lecky, F., Hawes, S., Silman, A., Macfarlane, G., et al., 2006. Predictors of persistent neck pain after whiplash injury. Emerg. Med. J. 23, 195–201.

Barnsley, L., Lord, S., Bogduk, N., 2002. The pathophysiology of whiplash. In: Malanga, G., Nadler, S. (Eds.), Whiplash, vol. 2. pp. 41–77.

Adapted Reflextherapy for pain – an alternative physiotherapy approach

Berry, G., 1999. Reflexology – when all else fails? CSP Congress. Poster Presentation, Birmingham.

Berry, G., 2003. Lower limb pain and dysfunction in adolescent boys and girls – clinical reasoning and treatment. Proceedings, World Congress Physical Therapy, Barcelona. Ref: SI-PO-0146.

Berry, G., 2007. Adapted Reflextherapy – a treatment for spinal pain and whiplash injury. FACT Focus on Alternative and Complementary Therapies 12 (1), 7.

Berry, G., 2007b. Adapted Reflextherapy in spinal pain including whiplash. Course Manual. Christie Hospital, Manchester, ongoing.

Breivik, H., Collett, B., Ventafridda, V., Cohen, R., Gallacher, D., 2005. Survey of chronic pain in Europe: Prevalence, impact on daily life, and treatment. Eur. J. Pain 10 (4), 287–333.

Butler, D., Moseley, L., 2003. Explain pain. NOI Group Publications, Adelaide, Australia.

Chien, A., Sterling, M., 2005. Central hypersensitivity in whiplash: Implications for physiotherapy assessment and management. Phys. Ther. Rev. 10, 237–245.

Chien, A., Eliav, E., Sterling, M., 2008. Hypoaesthesia occurs with sensory hypersensitivity in chronic whiplash – further evidence of a neuropathic condition. Man. Ther. 14 (2), 138–146.

Coderre, T., Katz, J., Vaccarino, A., Melzack, R., 1993. Contribution of central neuroplasticity to pathological pain: review of clinical and experimental evidence. Pain 52, 253–285.

Core Standards of Physiotherapy Practice, 2005. The Chartered Society of Physiotherapy, London.

Curatolo, M., Petersen-Felix, S., Arendt-Nielsen, L., Giani, C., Zbinden, A., Radanov, B., 2001. Central hypersensitivity in chronic pain after whiplash. Clin. J. Pain 17, 306–315.

Eliav, E., Herzberg, U., Ruda, M., Bennett, G., 1999. Neuropathic pain from an experimental neuritis of the rat sciatic nerve. Pain 83, 169–182.

Erdmann, A., Munglani, R., 2000. Advances in the management of spinal pain and radiofrequency techniques. In: Davidson, L. (Ed.), Whiplash. Bath, England, pp. 302–336.

Gracely, R., Lynch, S., Bennett, 1992. Painful neuropathy: altered central processing maintained dynamically by peripheral input. Pain 51, 175–194.

Greening, J., 2001. Minor nerve injury: an underestimated source of pain. The Olive Sands Memorial Lecture. In: Touch. Summer no 96, 7–12.

Greening, J., 2006. Workshop: clinical implications for clinicians treating patients with non-specific arm pain, whiplash and carpal tunnel syndrome. Man. Ther. 11, 171–172.

Guez, M., Hildingsson, C., Rosengren, L., Karlsson, K., Toolanen, G., 2003. Nervous tissue damage markers in cerebrospinal fluid after cervical spine injuries and whiplash trauma. J. Neurotrauma 20 (9), 853–858.

Hartling, L., Brison, R., Ardern, C., Pickett, W., 2001. Prognostic value of the Quebec Classification of whiplash-associated disorders. Spine 26 (1), 36–41.

Ingham, E., 2005. Stories the feet can tell thru' reflexology, Stories the feet have told thru' reflexology, 10th print. Ingham Publishing, Florida, USA.

Kahl, C., Cleland, J., 2005. Visual analogue scale, numeric pain rating scale and the McGill Pain Questionnaire: an overview of psychometric properties. Physical Therapies Reviews 10, 123–128.

Khan, S., Otter, S., Springett, K., 2006. The effects of reflexology on foot pain and quality of life in a patient with rheumatoid arthritis: A case report. Foot 16, 112–116.

Lund, I., Ge, Y., Yu, L., Uvnas-Moberg, K., Wang, J., Yu, C., et al., 2005. Repeat massage-like stimulation induces long-term effect on nociception: contribution of oxytocinergic mechanisms. Eur. J. Neurosci. 22 (6), 1553–1554.

Mackereth, P., Booth, K., Hillier, V., Caress, A., 2008. Reflexology and progressive muscle relaxation training for people with multiple sclerosis: a crossover trail. Complement. Ther. Clin. Pract. In press.

McVicar, A., Greenwood, C., Fewell, F., D'Arcy, V., Chandrasekharan, S., Alldridge, L., 2007. Evaluation of anxiety, salivary cortisol and melatonin secretion following reflexology treatment: A pilot study in health individuals. Complement. Ther. Clin. Pract. 13, 137–145.

Malanga, G., Nadler, S., 2002. Whiplash. Hanley & Belfus, Philadelphia.

Marchand, F., Perretti, M., McMahon, S., 2005. Role of the immune system in chronic pain. Nat. Rev. Neurosci. 6, 521–532.

Melzack, R., Wall, P., 1991. The challenge of pain. Penguin Books, Clays, London.

APPLICATIONS IN CLINICAL PRACTICE

Passatore, M., Roatta, S., 2006. Influence of sympathetic nervous system on sensorimotor function: whiplash associated disorder (WAD) as a model. Eur. J. Appl. Physiol. 98, 423–449.

Paterson, C., 1996. Measuring outcome in primary care: a patient-generated measure, MYMOP, compared to the SF-36 health survey. BMJ 312, 1016–1020.

Pauly, N., 2009. Nerve reflexology Level 1. Course Manual, International Association for Manual Neuro Therapy and Nerve Reflexology, MNT-NR (Feb).

Quinn, F., Baxter, G., Hughes, C., 2008. Complementary therapies in the management of low back pain: a survey of reflexologists. Complement. Ther. Med. 16 (1), 9–14.

Rothschild, B., 2000. The body remembers: The psychophysiology of trauma and trauma treatment. Norton, London.

Saab, C., Hains, B., 2008. Remote neuroimmune signalling: a long-range mechanism of nociceptive network plasticity. Trends Neurosci. 32 (2), 110–117.

Samuel, C.A, Campbell, I., Ebenezer, I., 2003. Reflexology in the management of pain. Pain management: is there a role for complementary medicine? 2 December. The Prince of Wales's Foundation for Integrated Health, London.

Scott, D., Jull, G., Sterling, M., 2005. Widespread sensory hypersensitivity is a feature of chronic whiplash associated disorder but not chronic idiopathic neck pain. Clin. J. Pain 21 (2), 175–181.

Stephenson, N.L.N., Dalton, J.A., 2003. Using reflexology for pain management. A review. J. Holist. Nurs. 21 (2), 179–191.

Sterling, M., Jull, G., 2003. Sensory hypersensitivity occurs soon after whiplash injury and is associated with poor recovery. Pain 104 (3), 509–517.

Sterling, M., Kenardy, J., 2006. The relationship between sensory and sympathetic nervous system changes and posttraumatic stress reaction following whiplash injury – a prospective study. J. Psychosom. Res. 60, 387–393.

Sterling, M., Jull, G., Vicenzino, B., Kenardy, J., Darnell, R., 2005. Physical and psychosocial factors predict outcome following whiplash injury. Pain 114 (1–2), 141–148.

Tiran, D., Chummun, H., 2005. The physiological basis of reflexology and its use as a potential diagnostic tool. Complement. Ther. Clin. Pract. 11, 58–64.

Tobin, A., 2000. Audit of a GP Practice based physiotherapy service. Wiltshire and Swindon Health Care NHS Trusts & Swindon and Marlborough NHS Trust, Sept.

Van Griensven, H., 2005. Pain in practice. Theory and treatment. Strategies for manual therapists. Butterworth Heinemann, London.

Watson, P.J., 1999. Psychosocial assessment. The emergence of a new fashion, or a new tool in physiotherapy for musculoskeletal pain. Physiotherapy 85 (10), 530–535.

Williamson, J., 1999. A guide to precision reflexology. Mark Allen, Wiltshire.

FURTHER READING

Byers, D., 2006. Better health with foot reflexology. Ingham Publishing, Florida, USA.

Gifford, L. (Ed.), 1998. Topical issues in pain: whiplash and management, fear-avoidance beliefs and behaviour. NOI Press, Falmouth, Cornwall.

Lett, A., 2000. ReflexZone Therapy for health professionals. Churchill Livingstone, London.

Marquardt, H., 2000. Reflexotherapy of the feet. Thieme Verlag, Germany.

Moore, A., Jackson, A., Jordan, H., Hammersley, S., Hill, J., Mercer, C., et al., 2005. Clinical guidelines for the physiotherapy management of whiplash associated disorder. Chartered Society of Physiotherapy, London.

USEFUL RESOURCES

Association of Chartered Physiotherapy in Reflextherapy (ACPIRT). Secretary: Christen Herbert, MCSP, 202 Childwall Road, Liverpool, L15 6UY; email: christenherbert@christen.f9.co.uk.

For further information regarding courses in AdRx run by the author contact: email jane@rosslaws.co.uk.

Adapted Reflextherapy for pain – an alternative physiotherapy approach

Adapting reflexology for cancer care

Peter Mackereth • Anita Mehrez
With contributions from Julia M. Williams •
Edwina Hodkinson

CHAPTER CONTENTS

ABSTRACT

For many people, advances in cancer treatment have afforded remission from the disease. Where this has not been possible, life may be extended with improved quality of symptom management. Reflexology can be a therapeutic and positive experience for patients and carers in cancer and palliative care settings. This chapter examines key issues in the provision of reflexology for people living with cancer. The content will focus on innovative, safe and skilled approaches to reflexology, including adaptation of techniques and skills.

KEY WORDS

Cancer, palliative and supportive care, myths, resilience, adaptations and carers.

INTRODUCTION

One in four people in the UK is likely to be affected by cancer at some time in their life and, for many, improvements in medical treatments mean that the disease will go into remission. In the UK a reduction of at least 20% of cancer deaths is expected in those under 75 years of age by 2010 (DoH, 2008). Cancer care has dramatically changed over the last three decades with an emphasis on early diagnosis and treatment, and an evidence-based approach to symptom management. Additionally, there is an international emphasis on improving lifestyles to reduce the impact of predisposing factors to cancer, with legislation and health campaigns focused on reducing smoking, obesity and abuse of alcohol and encouraging healthier diets and exercise. The role of reflexologists in assisting people making lifestyle changes is discussed in Chapter 13.

Cancer is not a single disease, but many, with different areas and tissues of the body affected. Diagnosis may follow investigation of unusual lumps, growths, persistent pain, and changes in weight or bleeding. Some cancers are difficult to diagnose and/or patients may be fearful of seeking medical advice. As the disease progresses, secondary growths, or metastases, may occur in other areas of the body. Treatment can include surgery, chemotherapy, radiotherapy, steroids and hormones, with some of these in combination (Watson et al. 2005). If the disease cannot be brought into remission, the focus of medical care is to support the patients to live well, based on the aims of palliative care, which:

1. affirms life and regards dying as a normal process
2. neither hastens nor postpones death
3. provides relief from pain and other symptoms
4. integrates psychological and spiritual aspects of patient care
5. offers a support system to help patients live as actively as possible until death
6. offers a support system to help the family cope during the patient's illness and in their own environment (Jeffrey 2003).

A European survey indicated that over 35% of people living with cancer will access complementary therapies, with high expectations of benefits (Molassiotis et al. 2006). When faced with a cancer diagnosis some patients may seek out 'cures' and can have unrealistic expectations of treatments. Therapists offering their services must be fully aware that under the Cancer Act, 1939, it is illegal to take sole responsibility for the treatment of people with cancer or to imply or make a promise of 'cure'. 'Healing' as distinct from 'curing' must be differentiated when engaging with clients about therapeutic outcomes. For example, a treatment might be a 'healing' experience, improve well-being and assisting with symptom management, but makes no discernible difference to disease progression (see Case Study 12.4).

REFLEXOLOGY AND RESILIENCE DURING THE CANCER JOURNEY

The term 'resilience' has been used to describe the ability of people to cope with major life stresses (Hunter 2001). A resilient individual will confront adversity and find a way of coping, surviving and even thriving (Garmezy 1991). The capacity to meet, cope with and overcome adversities can be developed and enhanced, given the right conditions and support. Moorey and Greer (1989), in their work with people who had received a cancer diagnosis, identified and classified the following coping styles:

• positive avoidance
• fighting spirit
• helpless/hopelessness

- anxious preoccupation
- stoical acceptance.

These styles may be perceived as negative but need not be adhered to rigidly; for example, positive avoidance may be appropriate when spending time being involved with pleasant things and not dwelling on worries or concerns. Stoically accepting one's situation can also be helpful; it is certainly a way of avoiding or containing anxiety. Anxious preoccupation (going over and over fears/worries) and/or feeling helpless and hopeless will undermine an individual's ability to cope and can be extremely overwhelming.

In contrast, the fighting spirit has been linked with survivorship, an approach to self-empowerment which is important and of great interest to patients, researchers, disease-specific support groups and therapists alike. This can be more complex than it first seems. For example, women with breast cancer, who have sought out radical and alternative means of staying well and fighting the disease, could be described as taking a heroine's path, although women whose cancers have progressed can feel devastated for 'failing' and guilty for not doing 'enough' or not doing it 'right' (Gray et al. 1998). Survival strategies such as buying and preparing large quantities of fresh fruit and vegetables for juicing and completely excluding 'junk food' may be proactive and positive, but making these changes can be very difficult. Participants in Sinding and Gray's (2005) study advocated a revised 'spunky' approach to cancer survivorship which embraces discussion of fears and concerns, living well, eating healthily, and engaging in therapies, such as reflexology, whilst even enjoying fun activities and 'naughty but nice' treats.

Reflexology can provide a nurturing source of support and comfort (see Fig. 12.1) for patients exhibiting these various coping styles. Those who are stoic or taking an avoidance stance may not be the first to turn to complementary therapies – and declining reflexology can be very empowering for them. Those in 'fighting spirit' mode may be clamouring to receive reflexology, while health professionals may refer patients who are anxious and preoccupied, or feeling helpless and hopeless, for much needed support. An understanding of coping styles informs our awareness of the varying responses to diagnosis and/or the challenges of treatment and can help therapists working in a cancer unit to accept when someone declines reflexology.

SAFETY, MYTHS AND FITNESS FOR PRACTICE

Reflexologists who specialise in treating patients with cancer need to consider their own resilience, as 'burnout' is a well-recognised phenomenon in cancer and hospice care (Isikhan et al. 2004). Burnout can lead us to distance ourselves from others, to feel physically and emotional unwell, exhausted and demotivated to work. Working with cancer patients can be emotionally challenging. Patients and their relatives need constant emotional support, which can be draining, and sometimes the work may cause therapists' personal experiences of cancer to be relived or revisited, such as recalling a patient who died or a family member with a similar disease. It is essential to safeguard one's practice and to incorporate strategies for self-protection, including taking time to reflect on practice experience, noticing personal uneasiness with different situations or tackling concerns which cause challenges at work.

Adapting reflexology for cancer care

Supervision, coaching, mentoring and debriefing sessions can be invaluable, as can reflecting on events and experiences (see Ch. 5). Reflexologists should make arrangements to receive complementary therapies for relaxation and respite, and to develop positive coping strategies to manage personal stress and maintain resilience (Mackereth & Carter 2006; Wilson et al. 2007).

Reflexology students and some health professionals may be aware of controversial opinions about the safety of reflexology for people living with cancer and its treatments. Despite some commonly held beliefs, there is no published evidence to suggest that cancer is a contraindication to reflexology. Indeed, it is more often the *therapist* rather than the *therapy* that is contraindicated. The UK National Curriculum for Reflexology now asserts that students require knowledge of cancer and its treatments, as well as the skills to adapt treatments safely (O'Hara 2006).

These concerns rest on the belief that reflexology may cause further tissue trauma and even spread cancer, especially in patients with lymphoedema, altered haematological states (i.e. neutropaenia and thrombocytopaenia), neuropathy, deep vein thrombosis and/or metastatic changes. The reflexologist can always engage in some gentle holding or consider working on the hands if the feet are not accessible. The belief that reflexology will 'spread cancer cells' is unfounded, given that blood circulation and lymphatic flow are stimulated by everyday activities of daily living, such as taking a bath or walking (Hodkinson 2001; Hodkinson et al. 2006). When lymphoedema is present, treatment may be avoided on the affected foot to prevent detrimental tissue pressure, although the non-lymphoedematous foot or hand can be treated (White 2006). Creative approaches to delivering reflexology are described below.

Perhaps the two most undeniable contraindications to reflexology in this client group are those who consciously decline treatment, and those who are unable to consent to treatment. Additionally, patients with resistant infection which may be transferred to the therapist or others may mean that skin-to-skin contact must be limited. It is essential that infection control policies and practices are adhered to at all times, including thorough hand washing and drying before and after contact with each and every patient. In clinical settings, strict adherence to hand washing techniques and the use of alcohol hand-rubbing solutions is closely monitored and subject to spot checks by hospital staff. The practitioner must also take care of his or her posture when providing treatment to patients in bed, in a wheelchair and/or when surrounded by equipment and carers, to avoid working at an awkward angle, which may cause discomfort, pain, injury or even repetitive strain (Pyves & Mackereth 2002).

Some reflexologists believe that handling the patients' feet and hands will cause them to become contaminated by the residue of cytotoxic drugs on the patients' skin. Cytotoxic drugs are metabolised by the liver and by-products are excreted in urine and faeces (Dougherty & Bailey 2001), so cross-contamination should not be of concern to reflexologists who do not handle the drugs or patients' body fluids. Also, there is no evidence of adverse reactions from reflexology for patients receiving chemotherapy. Indeed, the reduced anxiety, improvements in wellbeing, deep relaxation and decreased nausea and vomiting which result from reflexology treatment far outweigh the small risk of adverse reactions (Grealish et al. 2000; Stephenson & Weinrich 2000; Smith, 2002; Quattrin et al. 2006).

Radiotherapy treatment has also been considered a contraindication to receiving reflexology. However, since residual radioactive material is not

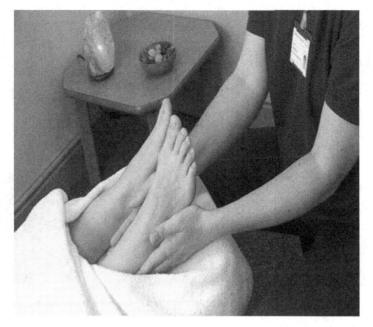

FIG. 12.1 Holding the feet, holding the person.

present in the body following radiotherapy treatment, reflexology is safe for both the patient and the therapist (Faithfull 2001). In the case of treatments and diagnostic procedures involving implanted radioactive material, careful adherence by the reflexologist to the strict rules of contact applied to medical and nursing staff, relatives (especially intimate partners) and carers will eliminate any need for concern.

The reflexologist who treats patients with cancer must take responsibility to remain fit and healthy enough to practice and should take care not to place vulnerable patients at risk from infection. Suppression of the immune system is a common consequence of cytotoxic chemotherapy, radiotherapy, high-dose steroids, blood/marrow transplantation or disease involvement of the bone marrow. If the reflexologist develops a sore throat, cold, influenza, diarrhoea, vomiting, or feels unwell, contact with immunocompromised patients should be avoided.

CREATIVE APPROACHES TO CLINICAL REFLEXOLOGY

Reflexology is one of the top three complementary therapies used in hospice and cancer care centres in the UK (Kohn 2002). Reflexology treatment can be given almost anywhere, in a specially equipped therapy room, at the patient's bedside in hospital, in the patient's home, or in a garden on a warm sunny day (Hodkinson et al. 2006) (Fig. 12.2). Informed consent, safety and comfort are essential tenets to providing reflexology to vulnerable individuals and it is essential to adapt the treatment appropriately.

The frequency and duration of reflexology treatments should be individualised and the reflexologist must be cautious so that treatment does not overtax the patient. Fatigue is a major problem for many patients, sometimes persisting for months or even years after completing treatment (Molassiotis et al.

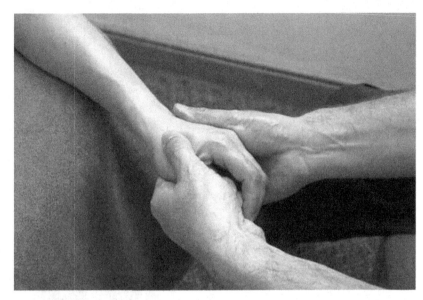

FIG. 12.2 Practitioner working at the bedside on the hand. *Photo courtesy of Katie Spruce BA (Hons), medical photographer, Christie Hospital NHS Trust, with permission.*

2007). Treatment duration may be as short as 15 minutes or up to 50 minutes, depending upon the patient's health, reaction to the session and the reason for undertaking it, but shorter, more frequent treatments may suit some patients (Figure 12.3). Treatment can be performed with the patient lying in a lateral position if this is the most comfortable. Breathless patients can rest their arms and head forward on several pillows on a fixed bed table which allows the lungs to expand and reduces pressure on the shoulder girdle. The quality of treatment and the tenderness of the touch are more important than adhering

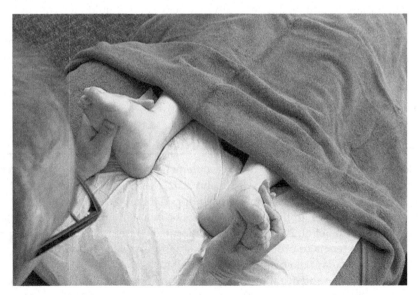

FIG. 12.3 Practitioner making contact with the feet. *Photo courtesy of Katie Spruce BA (Hons), medical photographer, Christie Hospital NHS Trust, with permission.*

Table 12.1 Creative approaches to adapting reflexology practice	
Techniques	**Brief descriptor**
Precision Reflexology Developed by Prue Miskin & Jan Williams	Gentle linking of specific reflexology points. Techniques can involve stillness and focus. Specific areas of the body such as the endocrine system and charkas of body are treated. Links can also involve bony structures and organs of the body
AirReflexology© Developed by Edwina Hodkinson & Barbara Cook	Involves combining reflexology theory and map to provide 'off the skin' or energy field reflexology
HypnoReflexology© Developed by Peter Mackereth & Paula Maycock	Deep relaxation techniques using breath work, pressure point work combined with hypnotherapy techniques, i.e. controlled use of the voice, safe space, and anchoring techniques to help with anxiety, needle phobia, pain and nausea
Creative Relaxation Reflexology (CRR) Barbara Cook	Combines gentle reflexology with creative imagery and visualisation
4-Hands Holding Reflexology (Mackereth et al. 2000)	Involves two qualified therapists working together with a patient. Treatments are usually shorter and can involve working the feet and hands together (see Fig. 12.4)

rigidly to a set time or to performing a complete treatment. Descriptors of examples of creative approaches to adapting reflexology practice are described briefly in Table 12.1, summarised from the work of colleagues and the authors of this chapter (Hodkinson et al. 2006) and several case studies are described in Case Studies 12.1–12.4. Specific techniques used for some of these patients are discussed in more detail in Chapters 13 and 14.

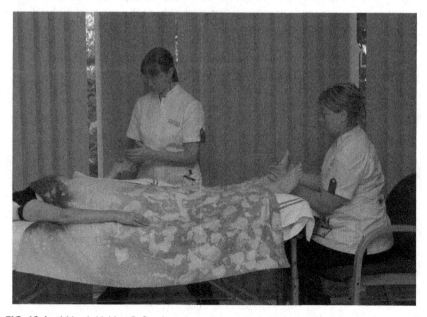

FIG. 12.4 4-Hands Holding Reflexology – two therapists combining hand and feet work.

Jason, aged 17, had a diagnosis of osteosarcoma. His condition required an above-knee amputation and following the operation he had difficulties with phantom limb pain and discomfort. His mother was present during his chemotherapy treatment. Jason talked about the family garden and greenhouse. The therapist offered to incorporate creative imagery into the treatment using the garden image and AirReflexology©.

The therapist first worked on the remaining right foot and left hand. She then used AirReflexology© over the physical shape of the missing foot in the position where it was 'lying' in his mind's eye. After the treatment, Jason said he could feel the presence of the therapist working over his absent limb and found it very comforting. His mother watched with fascination and asked if she could learn a simple technique to help him relax at home.

On subsequent chemotherapy sessions, Jason's mother learnt how to carry out simple hand reflexology, while the therapist attended to his right foot and provided AirReflexology© to the left missing limb (4-Hands Holding Reflexology).

CASE STUDY 12.2

Jeffrey, aged 57, was diagnosed with prostate cancer. During his recovery from radical surgery Jeffrey became terrified of needles and could not be cannulated for follow-up chemotherapy. He was angry at his inability to control the situation and to 'think away' his difficulty. This added to his distress. He withdrew his arm involuntarily at every attempt to cannulate, and treatment became impossible.

Jeffrey agreed to use hypnotherapy combined with reflexology (HypnoReflexology©) to help him with cannulation. Deep relaxation was achieved by using gentle pressure to the solar plexus reflex point of his hand combined with a guided breathing technique. After 2 minutes, Jeffrey stated he felt surprisingly calm and was ready to be cannulated. He was amazed when he was told it had already been successful. He continued to receive reflexology during the remaining cycles of chemotherapy. Jeffrey reported feeling empowered by his success and chose to learn self-hypnosis using hand reflexology points to support him in his recovery.

CASE STUDY 12.3

Penny, aged 67, had ovarian cancer and advanced disease. Whilst in hospital having withdrawal of ascites from her abdomen she was offered gentle reflexology combined with creative imagery. Towards the end of the treatment, Penny talked about an earlier visit from one of the medical staff who asked her if she would like to receive respite care at home or in a local hospice. Penny commented he was such a nice man but 'oh so serious'. She said, 'What I love about this treatment is how it feels, like a holiday from cancer … in a blissful state … cosseted and cuddled through my feet.'

> **CASE STUDY 12.4**
>
> Sarah was a terminally ill 25-year-old single mother with two small children who had chosen to spend her final weeks at home with her family. She was having two reflexology treatments weekly through a community outreach project. Sarah's mother, Sandra, would sit in the room whilst Sarah received her treatment and often fell asleep during the session. Sandra was then offered a reflexology treatment which enabled her to release her emotions and the tears flowed. Sarah expressed relief that her mother was able to show how she was feeling and they embraced each other ... and the therapist. Sandra continued to access reflexology following Sarah's death.

CARING FOR CARERS

Carers, the relatives and friends of patients going through investigation, treatment and imparting of prognosis (Thomas et al. 2002) can become deeply distressed, especially when sitting with them during these procedures. A diagnosis of cancer is frightening and stressful, not only for the immediate family, but also for close friends and work colleagues. It can have a profound impact on personal relationships and affect people's ability to talk openly about feelings, fears and concerns. Carers may have a strong desire to protect the patient from the full impact of the disease and its treatment; even to the point that they want health professionals to speak to them before the patient, and providing daily care, especially if the patient remains at home, can be physically and emotionally draining in the extreme, causing them to neglect their own needs. Alongside these concerns are the pressures to cope with family demands, work and financial concerns.

Henwood's study (1998) revealed that 51% of carers had suffered a physical injury and 52% had been treated for stress-related illness since the onset of care provision, while Payne et al. (1999) reported psychosocial distress and high levels of strain related to care-giving. Carers also report life restrictions, emotional distress and perceived lack of support, reduced energy levels and high anxiety (Aranda & Haynman-White 2001). Reflexology can be extremely beneficial for carers in these situations, although they may need to be convinced that they deserve a treatment, often feeling that the patient 'needs it more than they do'. It can, however, be very relaxing for the patient to watch their carer receiving reflexology and being 'permitted' to take time out and care for themselves (Campbell et al. 2006) (see Case Study 12.4).

Providing supportive reflexology at a time of great stress and physical challenge can give carers time to recuperate, relax, to receive attention as valued contributors to patient care and to assist with sustaining resilience (Mackereth & Carter 2006). If they wish to continue with reflexology after the death of their loved one, then this can provide positive help for the grieving process. Carers may want to be involved in providing reflexology to their loved ones (see Case Study 12.1), but this must be in accordance with the patient's wishes and the carer must feel comfortable about doing the treatment. Teaching a skill requires sensitive handling, particularly when the carer is keen to 'get it right' for his or her loved one at a crucial time. Personal experience of a gentle reflexology treatment helps the carer to appreciate appropriate pressure, movements and pace. For more information about teaching carers, see Chapter 10.

CONCLUSION

Reflexology has the potential to be a valuable intervention for both patients and their carers during the cancer treatment and care journey. Reflexology can assist in maintaining well-being during challenging cancer treatments, as well as providing comfort and support with symptoms and side effects which are difficult to treat. Reflexology is not a 'cure' but can provide a 'healing space' – an opportunity to take a break from being a 'cancer patient' or carer. The skilled therapist requires knowledge of cancer and its treatments; an awareness and sensitivity to the needs of patient and carers, as well as a willingness to adapt to unique situations as they arise. Support and supervision are crucial to avoid burnout and to provide responsive, considered and accountable care. See Box 12.1 for key recommendations when working in cancer care.

> **BOX 12.1 Recommendation for best practice in cancer care**
>
> ■ Be aware of differing ways in which patients and carers respond to and cope with diagnosis and the challenges of treatment.
>
> ■ Be informed about cancer, its treatments and side effects, and sources of information, and support collaboratively with healthcare professionals to ensure treatments take account of health concerns, effects of treatment and need for careful observation.
>
> ■ Acknowledge limitations and seek skills in adapting reflexology treatments to ensure safety, comfort and effectiveness.
>
> ■ Offer short and gentle sessions for patients with fatigue and/or undergoing chemotherapy or radiotherapy.
>
> ■ Consider how to involve and empower patients (and carers), e.g. teaching self-help techniques with skilled supervision.
>
> ■ Evaluate, reflect upon and develop best practice, whilst being mindful of one's own resilience and need for support in this challenging work.
>
> ■ Gather and review research evidence to inform reflexology practice within cancer care settings.

REFERENCES

Aranda, S.K., Hayman-White, K., 2001. Home caregivers of the person with advanced cancer. An Australian perspective. Cancer Nurs. 24 (4), 300–307.

Campbell, G., Mackereth, P.A., Sylt, P., 2006. In: Mackereth, P., Carter, A. (Eds.), Massage & bodywork: adapting therapies for cancer care. Churchill Livingstone, London.

Department of Health (DoH), 2008. Cancer reform strategy. Department of Health. www.dh.gov.uk/publications.

Dougherty, L., Bailey, C., 2001. Chemotherapy. Cancer nursing: care in context. Blackwell Science, Oxford.

Faithfull, S., 2001. Radiotherapy. Cancer nursing: care in context. Blackwell Science, Oxford.

Garmezy, N., 1991. Resilience in children's adaptation to negative life events and stressed environments. Pediatr. Ann. 20, 459–466.

Gray, R., Fitch, M., Greenberg, M., Hampson, A., Doherty, M., Labrecque,

1998. The information needs of well long-term survivors of breast cancer. Patient Educ. Couns. 33 (3), 245–255.

Grealish, L., Lomasney, A., Whiteman, B., 2000. Foot massage: a nursing intervention to modify the distressing symptoms of pain and nausea in patients hospitalised with cancer. Cancer Nurs. 23 (3), 237–243.

Henwood, M., 1998. Ignored or invisible? Carers' experience of the NHS. Carers' National Association.

Hodkinson, E., 2001. The benefits of reflexology in palliative care. Reflexions. J. Assoc. Reflexologists 63, 27.

Hodkinson, E., Cook, B., Mackereth, P.A., 2006. Creative approaches to reflexology. In: Mackereth, P., Carter, A. (Eds.), Massage & bodywork: adapting therapies for cancer care. Churchill Livingstone, London.

Hunter, A., 2001. A cross-cultural comparison of resilience in adolescents. J. Pediatr. Nurs. 16 (3), 172–179.

Isikhan, V., Comez, T., Danis, Z., 2004. Job stress and coping strategies in health care professionals working with cancer patients. Eur. J. Oncol. Nurs. 8, 234–244.

Jeffrey, D., 2003. What do we mean by psychosocial care in palliative care? In: Williams, M.L. (Ed.), Psychosocial issues in cancer care. Oxford University Press, Oxford.

Kohn, M., 2002. Complementary therapies in cancer care. Macmillan Cancer Relief, London.

Mackereth, P., Carter, A., 2006. Nurturing resilience: touch therapies in palliative care. J Holistic Healthcare 3 (1), 24–28.

Mackereth, P., Pyves, G., 2002. Working safely. In: Mackereth, P., Tiran, D. (Eds.), Clinical reflexology: a guide for health professionals. Churchill Livingstone, Edinburgh.

Mackereth, P., Campbell, G., Norman, M., Knight, J., 2000. Introducing 4 hands holding: many hands make profound work. Cahoots 72, 36–38.

Molassiotis, A., Cawthorn, A., Mackereth, P.A., 2006. Complementary and alternative therapies. In: Kearney, N., Richardson, A. (Eds.), Nursing patients with cancer: principles and practice. Churchill Livingstone, London.

Molassiotis, A., Sylt, P., Diggins, H., 2007. The management of cancer-related fatigue after chemotherapy: a randomized controlled trial. Complement. Ther. Med. 15, 228–237.

Moorey, S., Greer, S., 1989. Psychological therapy for patients with cancer: a new approach. Heinemann, Oxford.

O'Hara, C.S., 2006. Core curriculum for reflexology. Douglas Barry, London.

Payne, S., Smith, S.P., Dean, S., 1999. Identifying the concerns of informal carers in palliative care. Palliat. Med. 13 (1), 37–44.

Quattrin, R., Zanini, A., Buchini, S., Turello, D., Annunziata, M.A., Vidotti Colombatti, A., et al., 2006. Use of reflexology foot massage to reduce anxiety in hospitalized cancer patients in chemotherapy treatment: methodology and outcomes. J. Nurs. Manag. 14, 96–105.

Sinding, C., Gray, R., 2005. Active aging – spunky survivorship? Discourses and experiences of the years beyond breast cancer. J. Aging Studies 19, 147–161.

Smith, G., 2002. A randomised controlled clinical trial of reflexology in breast cancer patients, to reduce fatigue resulting from radiotherapy to the breast & chest wall. Unpublished PhD thesis, University of Liverpool.

Stephenson, N.L.N., Weinrich, S.P., 2000. The effects of foot reflexology on anxiety and pain in patients with breast and lung cancer. Oncol. Nurs. Forum 27 (1), 67–72.

Thomas, C., Morris, S.M., Hanman, J.C., 2002. Companions through cancer: the care given by informal carers in cancer contexts. Soc. Sci. Med. 54 (4), 529–544.

Watson, M., Lucas, C., Hoy, A., Back, I., 2005. Oxford handbook of palliative care. Oxford University Press, Oxford.

White, C., 2006. Managing lymphoedema. In: Mackereth, P., Carter, A. (Eds.), Massage & bodywork: adapting therapies for cancer care. Churchill Livingstone, London.

Wilson, K., Ganley, A., Mackereth, P., Rowswell, V., 2007. Subsidised complementary therapies for staff and volunteers at a regional cancer centre: a formative study. Eur. J. Cancer Care 16, 291–299.

FURTHER READING

Kubler Ross, E., 1969. On death and dying. Touch Stone, New York.

Tavares, M., 2003. National Guidelines for the Use of Complementary Therapies in Supportive and Palliative Care. The Prince of Wales' Foundation for Integrated Health, London.

USEFUL ADDRESSES

National Association of Complementary Therapists in Hospice and Palliative Care 32 Milner Road, Selly Park, Birmingham, B29 7RQ
Tel: 0121 472 4987

Teenage Cancer Trust
Kirkman House, Kirkman Place, 54a Tottenham Court Road, London, W1P 9RF
Tel: 0207 436 2877
Fax: 0207 637 4302
E-mail:tct@teencancer.bdx.co.uk
Website: http://www.teencancer.org

Macmillan Cancer Relief Macmillan Fund
15–19 Britten Street, London, SW3 TZ
Tel: 0207 352 7811

Cancer Backup
3 Bath Place, Rivington Street, London, EC2A 3JR
Tel: 0207 613 2121

Marie Curie Cancer Care
28 Belgrave Square, London, SW1X 8QG
Tel: 0207 235 3325

Reflexology and withdrawal from addictive substances: a focus on smoking cessation

13

Paula Maycock • Peter Mackereth

ABSTRACT

In this chapter we explore how reflexology can help to support an individual through the challenging transition to being and sustaining a smoke/drug/alcohol-free state. Reflexology, while not a substitute for evidence-based addiction interventions, can be a potent vehicle for a client in contemplating, seeking and gaining a healthier perspective on life. Although the broader issues of addiction are examined briefly, this chapter focuses on how to assist a client with smoking cessation.

KEY WORDS

Smoking, reflexology, alcohol, drugs, cravings, change and support.

INTRODUCTION

Comprehensive history taking at the first reflexology appointment should include routine questions about lifestyle, including diet and nutrition, smoking, alcohol consumption and use of other substances. Perhaps not all practitioners would feel comfortable discussing these aspects, but a good awareness of recommended evidence-based strategies and agencies to support clients making lifestyle changes is fundamental to good practice. Practitioners should develop their knowledge about smoking cessation and drug and alcohol dependence, but this starts from within and may be influenced by values, attitudes and personal and professional experience.

In considering the role of reflexology in supporting individuals who wish to make lifestyle changes, it is important to be clear that this intervention is not a substitute for high-quality smoking cessation/drug and alcohol advisory/support services. There is, however, good evidence for reflexology being a valuable touch therapy for creating deep relaxation, assistance with anxiety reduction and a safe place for disclosure of worries and concerns (see Chs 2 and 6).

ADDICTIVE SUBSTANCES

Addiction has been defined as the 'uncontrolled compulsive use of a substance, person, thought or behaviour for the purpose of changing a person's emotional state, regardless of any potential consequences' (Wager & Cox 2009:1). Use of addictive substances has no race, religion, gender, sexuality or age boundary. Assumptions are often made that 'addicts' are hopeless individuals, who rarely accept help and need to be someone else's problem (ANSA 1997).

The reasons for onset of substance misuse are complex and varied. Introduction to the various substances may be associated with pleasure-seeking, risk-taking and peer pressure. Certain behaviours, habits and use of noxious substances often begin as a means of short-term coping with anxiety, stressful life events and ongoing psychological concerns, offering a temporary 'high', to pacify or even create a sense of numbness to concerns and challenging situations. However, in the long term, the continued and/or excessive use of these substances seriously compromises an individual's physical and mental health and well-being. There are also well-documented cases of harm with a single exposure (e.g. Ecstasy).

When addiction takes hold, unfulfilled cravings can cause an individual to behave erratically and to take risks in seeking the desired substance. Addiction which spirals out of control can lead to loss of employment, relationship breakdown, homelessness, self-harm, severe illness and even loss of life (Hunkeler et al. 2001; Lavikainen & Lintonen, 2009). Additionally, when the substance is an illegal drug or the person has no funds to finance the habit, the only option may be to turn, in desperation, to crime. As a consequence, harm to others and their property may lead to contact with the police and even imprisonment (ANSA 1997).

The burden of addiction to society and amongst individuals can be like an iceberg, with much of the problem hidden below the surface. An elderly person with arthritis living alone may combine painkillers with increasing amounts of alcohol to get through the day. An overworked business executive may increase consumption of both alcohol and cigarettes to the point where breathlessness on exertion occurs or important appointments are missed due to 'hangovers'.

Withdrawal from addictive substances, whether optional or enforced, can leave an uncomfortable, empty space, with various physical and psychological reactions (Table 13.1). Some effects are short-term, reaching their peak after a few days; other effects last for weeks or can become chronic. The duration for

Table 13.1	*Examples of withdrawal effects*
Alcohol	Sweating, insomnia, nausea, vomiting, hallucination and seizures
Caffeine	Irritability, loss of drive/motivation, fatigue, headaches, inability to concentrate and nausea
Cannabis	Loss of appetite, inability to sleep, anxiety, headache, nausea, paranoia, irritability and even aggression
Crack/cocaine	Anger, intense cravings of increasing strength, low mood and depression, agitation, nausea, vomiting and the shakes
Benzodiazepines	Anxiety, panic, insomnia, depression, jumpiness, dizziness, tremor, muscle pain, sweating, palpitations, poor memory and inability to concentrate
Tobacco	Irritability, aggression, low mood/depression, restlessness, increased appetite, light-headedness and waking at night
Opiates	Sweating, nausea and vomiting, diarrhoea, abdominal cramps, muscle aches, increase in heart and respiratory rate and raised blood pressure
Ashton 2005; Wager & Cox 2009	

which substances remain in the body varies from one person to another and between substances. For example, alcohol may still be present in the bloodstream and affect behaviour for 7 or more hours after consumption, and nicotine can take up to 48 hours to be completely excreted from the body (Ratner et al. 2004; Heck 2006).

Numerous local and national government-funded and voluntary support groups and specialist organisations exist to support individuals with substance misuse (see Useful Resources). In complementary therapy centres there are golden opportunities for practitioners to encourage and support smoking cessation, and for appropriately trained therapists to assist with drug and alcohol withdrawal programmes. In clinics where a variety of complementary therapies are available, an integrated approach may be appropriate, such as combining reflexology with hypnotherapy or acupuncture (see below). Evidence suggests that auricular acupuncture and clinical hypnotherapy are useful interventions for people wanting to stop smoking or to withdraw from drug and alcohol dependency (Ahijevych et al. 2000; White et al. 2000).

FOCUS ON SMOKING CESSATION

Since English legislation to ban smoking in 'enclosed and partially enclosed spaces' came into effect in 2007, it has become more difficult for smokers to 'light up' in public and even in some private spaces. Similar legislation has been introduced or is being considered in numerous countries around the world, and national and international campaigns to reduce the use of tobacco products have been widely instigated. Easier access to smoking cessation advice and support, increased engagement with young people, pregnant mothers and other hard-to-reach groups has received the support and funding of governments in many countries. Disturbingly, however, there is evidence of increasing tobacco use in the Third World as Western countries start to reduce tobacco consumption, and a high incidence of illegal trafficking in tobacco products, which are often adulterated with even more noxious substances and commonly linked to criminal activities (DoH 2008; WHO 2008).

Nicotine differs from other addictive substances, because users do not have immediately obvious effects of cognitive impairment which is often witnessed with other substances, so the problems associated with consent do not usually apply. Nicotine produces widespread nervous system effects, stimulating the release of adrenaline (epinephrine), noradrenaline (norepinephrine) and dopamine, vasopressin, serotonin, arginine, γ-aminobutyric acid, beta endorphins and other neurotransmitters in the body (Hurt et al. 2009). The effects of these changes may disguise or exacerbate underlying health conditions and affect the outcome of medical treatment. Nicotine may also be mixed with other drugs, either directly (e.g. cannabis) or taken concurrently with substances such as alcohol or cocaine. These combinations may interfere with the presentation of symptoms associated with physical and psychological imbalance.

Tobacco dependence should be viewed as a 'chronic' medical condition often requiring repeated intervention and numerous attempts to stop (Fiore et al. 2008). In the United States, 70% of smokers would like to stop smoking, nearly half of these attempting to stop on an annual basis (Hurt et al. 2009). In the UK, statistics for tobacco use vary geographically and between social class, age and gender, with up to 26% of manual workers smoking routinely (DoH 2008). The possibility is high that many clients seeking reflexology will be smokers, so supporting clients to stop smoking makes sound health practice, as well as good business sense. Nicotine replacement therapies (NRTs) and other well-researched medical treatments are the foundation of smoking cessation intervention (Lancaster et al. 2000).

ASSISTING PEOPLE DURING WITHDRAWAL

Tobacco, drugs and alcohol are major causes of preventable illness, injuries and death (DoH 2004), and clinical reflexologists can play a complementary, rather than an alternative, role in assisting individuals to manage and withdraw from addictive substances. This requires an understanding of addiction, the effects of withdrawal and a willingness to set aside assumptions and judgements about clients and why and how they became addicted. Substance misuse can create challenges for reflexologists to provide safe and sensitive treatment. For example, since many substances impair cognitive function or cause intoxication, particular care should be taken with setting boundaries between the client and the therapist, who is at liberty to stipulate that she or he wishes only to work with clients who are not under the active influence of drugs. Consent to treatment is essential, and therapists should be mindful of the alterations in social behaviour and inability to give informed consent to treatment which can result from substance misuse (see Ch. 4). Therapists may consider working within a group practice in a specialist centre with professional drug and alcohol workers on site. Working alone, particularly in this area of practice, may compromise a practitioner's safety.

THE ROLE OF REFLEXOLOGY

The 2006 survey by Sood et al. of 1175 smokers in the USA indicated that 27% had previously used one or more complementary therapies to help them to stop smoking, and 67% were interested in future use, with massage and relaxation being two of the top five choices. Therapeutic touch can be a valuable contribution to sustain engagement in the process of smoking cessation treatment. Hernandez-Reif et al. (1999) undertook a study (n=20) in which self-massage was taught to assist with reducing withdrawal symptoms and to facilitate adherence to treatment programmes.

The authors completed a national training programme of brief interventions for smoking cessation (NICE 2006) and a course in assessing whether clients are suitable for nicotine replacement therapies. Having received feedback from patients that reflexology helped with stopping smoking, they established a smoking cessation service within a hospital setting, offering complementary therapies, advice, support and conventional nicotine replacement therapies (NRTs) (Maycock & Mackereth 2009). The service is free at the point of delivery and available to patients, carers and staff. Referral rates are increasing all the time with more than twenty clients attending each week for advice and support (Maycock & Mackereth 2009) (see Fig. 13.1).

Clinical reflexologists who have developed the appropriate knowledge and skills to become competent and confident to treat clients withdrawing from tobacco, drugs and alcohol can play a valuable part in this area of healthcare. As with all clinical specialities, it is essential to audit and evaluate services and practice, and to use evidence or become involved in research projects to refine practice and improve outcomes.

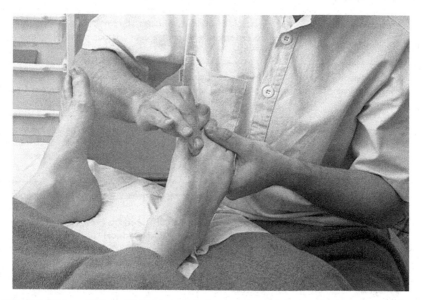

FIG. 13.1 Photo courtesy of Katie Spruce BA (Hons), medical photographer, Christie Hospital NHS Trust, with permission.

BEHAVIOURAL CHANGE MODEL

As a starting point for developing reflexology practice in this clinical area it is useful to consider a model to provide a workable framework for clinical care. An approach to behaviour change – the 'transtheoretical stages of change model' (Prochaska & DiClemente 1983) – has been utilised within health promotion and can be adapted for use in reflexology practice (Table 13.2). There are five crucial stages centred on the individual client's own decision-making processes. A client may have attended for reflexology for various reasons, and stopping smoking is unlikely to be the primary reason. The reflexologist can nurture the client with a view to initiating behavioural changes, which have demonstrable implications for longer-term health and well-being. Including smoking and alcohol consumption within the initial history-taking opens the door to a potential conversation on the subject, either at the first or a subsequent appointment, and may motivate the client to take steps to withdraw from smoking.

It may be useful to include the following questions in routine history taking:

- Do you use tobacco? If 'Yes' in what form, e.g. cigarettes, pipe, cigars, chewing tobacco, bubble tube? How many do you smoke a day? How soon after waking do you smoke?
- For how long have you used tobacco? What do you remember about the motivation/reasons for starting?
- To what extent do you want to stop smoking? What would be your main reasons for doing so?

Table 13.2 *The transtheoretical stages of change model and reflexology*

Stages	Role of the reflexologist
1. Precontemplation – I have no plans to change my smoking behaviour	Seed the possibility of change by: ○ including information in leaflets/introductions on support available to all clients wishing to be smoke free ○ record smoking history/status as a standard part of reflexology practice
2. Contemplation – I may consider planning to change my smoking	○ be open to discussing a client's 'contemplations' ○ be interested and provide encouragement about contemplation, e.g. are you still thinking about becoming smoke free?
3. Preparation – I will change my smoking in the next month	○ explore what support the client needs from the therapist, e.g. information on local smoking cessation services ○ explain how reflexology may assist in maintenance of well being during the withdrawal process
4. Action – I have started to reduce my smoking and have obtained Nicotine Replacement Therapy	○ teach self reflexology techniques, e.g. work hand reflex points for relaxation ○ confirm correct use of NRT products (refer to Smoking Cessation Specialist for further advice)
5. Maintenance – I have not smoked for the last 3 months	○ acknowledge and celebrate success ○ review self-help work and offer top-ups to maintain ongoing success

Adapted from Prochaska & DiClemente 1983.

- Have you stopped before? For how long? What did you use to assist you?
- Do any of your close family or friends smoke? Would they be interested in receiving support to stop?
- Would you like to know how reflexology might help you with smoking cessation?

Clients need to trust the therapist in order to feel able to disclose details about themselves that they may not have revealed to others. Contemplation may not be revealed at the first session. There is often a great sense of shame about the addiction, so trust needs to be built up (see Case Study 13.1). Offering a programme of six to ten sessions provides a regular nurturing and therapeutic space for rapport to develop. For a smoker, who may be hesitant about changing behaviour, the process can begin with tentative exploratory steps. Compassion and self-awareness on the part of the client is essential to this journey. It is useful to have an understanding of the original and current trigger to tobacco use, as well as the possible strategies that the individual might use, now or in the future, to maintain a smoke-free life.

CASE STUDY 13.1

Joan, aged 45 years, was awaiting surgery and feeling very anxious. During her third reflexology session she revealed that she felt ashamed about continuing to smoke 15 cigarettes a day (although she had told her GP that she only smoked 2–3 a day). Joan had been prescribed NRT lozenges to replace her 'occasional' cigarette but she had not opened them.

The therapist, trained in smoking cessation work, suggested that, rather than stopping completely, Joan could reduce her smoking by replacing alternate cigarettes with an NRT lozenge, and that she should continue to receive reflexology weekly. By the sixth session of reflexology Joan had completely replaced her cigarettes with lozenges. Six months later she had recovered well from the surgery and kept a packet of NRT lozenges in her handbag for support.

How might therapies such as reflexology help to ease the smoking cessation journey? It can be argued that reflexology provides essential time for clients to relax, receive nurturing touch and feel comfortable to disclose a dependency or to consider embarking on the challenging journey of change. At the root of the collaborative work for both the client and the therapist is an acknowledgement of the challenge confronting them as they strive to become smoke/drug/alcohol free. Reflexology can help to 'refill' the person to feel whole again in a positive and hopeful way, providing a choice to do something different to feel pleasure, feel alive and be in control. Teaching self-help work on hand reflex points can augment the weekly reflexology sessions (see Case Study 13.2).

CASE STUDY 13.2

Robert, aged 55 years, had oral cancer and had been admitted to hospital for both chemotherapy and radiotherapy. He had drunk alcohol and smoked since he was 16 years old. With no access to alcohol he was going out of the ward for 2–3 cigarettes up to 15 times a day, including during the night. Robert had

---

noticed that he had become more anxious and found it difficult to cope when he required needles to be inserted for his chemotherapy.

Reflexology was successfully used to assist with reducing the needle anxiety and Robert also reported a reduction in cravings for cigarettes for the remainder of the days on which treatment was given. He was eager to learn some hand reflexology to use at night when his cravings were at their worst. The therapists also encouraged Robert to use his NRT inhalator to maintain nicotine levels. Within a week Robert was cigarette free.

The authors, who are experienced reflexologists and qualified hypnotherapists, have developed an approach to treating clients wishing to stop smoking in which a synergistic combination of reflexology and hypnotherapy techniques are used (Hodkinson et al. 2006). This integrative package known as HypnoReflexology© provides a therapeutic space to identify the client's resources and appropriate and acceptable strategies to manage the journey (see Case Study 13.3). Other members of the smoking cessation team who are not hypnotherapists combine creative imagery and relaxation skills with reflexology, also with good effect (Maycock & Mackereth 2009).

CASE STUDY 13.3

Vanessa attended a smoking cessation drop-in clinic offering reflexology, hypnotherapy and acupuncture after her son had challenged her about her smoking habits when he saw a televised government campaign encouraging people to stop smoking. During her first session Vanessa became deeply relaxed with a combination of reflexology and hypnotherapy (HypnoReflexology©). She recalled that she had been an isolated teenager desperate to be a part of a crowd, which had resulted in her trying her first cigarette. During the session Vanessa recognised that she no longer needed cigarettes to be the person she is now. When asked who she felt was her supporter, Vanessa immediately visualised her son saying, 'I am so proud of you Mum, going to university and stopping smoking'. Vanessa chose to use this image and his words to strengthen her resolve to be smoke free. Vanessa stopped smoking after three sessions and was still smoke-free 6 months later.

The approach taken by the authors in clinical practice is one of combining effective use of pharmacological agents with supportive and complementary care. It is important to stress that compliance with NRT products (and other pharmacological interventions) is best facilitated by skilled smoking cessation advisors and combined with strategies to reduce stress and anxiety. It is essential to network with outside agencies in order to gain information about local support services that clients and therapists working in this field should explore. Most of the national agencies have local groups (see Useful Resources); public libraries hold valuable information on smaller groups in their locality. In the community, local smoking cessation advisors, alcohol and drug advisors/ counsellors, GPs, practice nurses, pharmacists and occupational health advisors are key professionals with whom to engage and from whom to gather information. Additionally, mentoring and training from smoking cessation specialists is essential in maintaining good clinical practice. Working with clients who use addictive substances can be extremely challenging for therapists and it is imperative that all therapists in this field engage in regular clinical supervision via a peer group or in a one-to-one session with a skilled therapist (Mackereth 2001).

CONCLUSION

It is hoped that readers will now take time to consider whether, and how, assisting clients with smoking cessation could become a part of their normal reflexology practice. Practice points for clinical reflexologists are summarised in Box 13.1. Supporting someone who wishes to become smoke free or working with those with other addictive behaviours can be incredibly rewarding, often leading clients to spread the word to family and friends, who may then self-refer for help to change their behaviour.

BOX 13.1 Practice points for clinical reflexologists

- It is essential to develop appropriate skills and to obtain support and supervision to offer clinical reflexology to clients withdrawing from smoking, drugs and alcohol usage.
- When providing home treatments insist on working in a smoke-free space – this is your right under UK law and acts as a role model for protecting one's own health.
- Be open, interested and supportive to clients, listening to them and assisting them to explore smoking and other addictive behaviours.
- Reflexology has the potential to provide a safe environment for disclosure regarding tobacco/drug/alcohol dependency.
- Be able to direct clients and/or seek out information about local services and national help lines (see Useful Resources).
- If the client is already using NRT or other medical interventions to manage cravings, reflexology can be valuable as a means of support and maintaining compliance.
- Insist that clients do not arrive for their reflexology appointments under the influence of drugs or alcohol.
- Reflexology is not an alternative but a complementary intervention to support evidence-based practice in smoking cessation/alcohol/drug-dependency programmes.
- Consider further training in creative imagery, relaxation skills or clinical hypnotherapy to support clients.

REFERENCES

Ahijevych, K., Yerardi, R., Nedilsky, N., 2000. Descriptive outcomes of the American Lung Association of Ohio Hypnotherapy Smoking Cessation Program. Int. J. Clin. Exp. Hypn. 48 (4), 374–1338.

Ashton, C.H., 2005. Diagnosis and management of benzodiazepines dependence. Curr. Opin. Psychiatry 18 (3), 249–255.

Association of Nurses in Substance Abuse (ANSA), 1997. Substance use: guidance on good clinical practice for specialist nurses. Pinpoint Communication, Kingston-Upon-Thames.

Department of Health (DoH), 2004. Summary of intelligence on tobacco. HMSO, London.

Department of Health (DoH), 2008. Excellence in tobacco control: 10 high-impact changes to achieve tobacco control. www.dh.gov.uk/publication.

Fiore, M., Baker, T., Jaen, C., Bailey, W., Benowitz, N., Curry, S., et al., 2008. Clinical practice guideline – 2008 update. US Department of Health & Human Services, Rockville, MD.

Heck, A., 2006. Review of alcohol clearance in humans. Alcohol 15 (3), 147–160.

Hernandez-Reif, M., Field, T., Hart, S., 1999. Smoking cravings are reduced by self-massage. Prevent. Med. 28 (1), 29–31.

Hodkinson, E., Cook, B., Mackereth, P., 2006. Creative approaches to reflexology. In: Mackereth, P., Carter, A. (Eds.), Massage & bodywork: adapting therapies for cancer care. Elsevier Science, London.

Hunkeler, E.M., Hung, Y.Y., Rice, D.P., Weisner, C., Hu, T., 2001. Alcohol consumption patterns and health care costs in an HMO. Drug Alcohol Depend. 64 (2), 181–190.

Hurt, R.D., Ebbert, J.O., Hays, J.T., McFadden, D.D., 2009. Treating tobacco dependence in a medical setting. A Journal For Cancer Clinicians 59, 314–326.

Lancaster, T., Stead, L., Silagy, C., Sowden, A., 2000. Effectiveness of interventions to help people stop smoking: findings from the Cochrane Library. BMJ 5 (321), 355–358 (7257).

Lavikainen, H.M., Lintonen, T.P., 2009. Alcohol use in adolescence: identifying harms related to teenager's alcohol drinking. J. Substance Use 14, 39–48.

Mackereth, P., 2001. Clinical supervision. In: Rankin-Box, D. (Ed.), The nurses' handbook of complementary therapies. Churchill Livingstone, London.

Maycock, P., Mackereth, P., 2009. Helping smokers to stop. Int. Therapist 86, 18–19.

National Institute for Health and Clinical Excellence (NICE), 2006. Brief interventions and referral for smoking cessation. National Institute for Health and Clinical Excellence, London.

Prochaska, J.O., DiClemente, C., 1983. Stages and processes of self-change of smoking: toward an integrated model of change. J. Consult. Clin. Psychol. 51, 390–395.

Ratner, A., Johnson, J., Richardson, C., Bottorff, J., Moffat, B., Mackay, M., et al., 2004. Efficacy of smoking cessation intervention for elective-surgical patients. Res. Nurs. Health 27, 148–161.

Sood, A., Ebbert, J.O., Sood, R., Stevens, S.R., 2006. Complementary treatments for tobacco cessation: a survey. Nicotine Tob. Res. 8 (6), 767–771.

Wager, K., Cox, S., 2009. Auricular acupuncture & addiction: mechanisms, methodology and practice. Elsevier Science, London.

White, A.R., Rampas, H., Ernst, E., 2000. Acupuncture for smoking cessation. Cochrane Database Syst. Rev. 2, CD000009.

World Health Organization (WHO), 2008. Report on the global tobacco epidemic – the MPOWER package. World Health Organization, Geneva.

FURTHER READING

Miller, N. (Ed.), 2004. Comprehensive handbook of drug and alcohol addiction. University of Newcastle. www.benzo.org.uk.

Miller, W., Rollinick, S., 2002. Motivational interviewing: Preparing people for change, second ed. Guildford Press, New York.

Tomlinson, L., Maycock P., Mackereth, P. Helping a person go smoke-free: an integrative hypnotherapy approach. In: Cawthorn A., Mackereth, P. (Eds.) Integrated hypnotherapy. Elsevier Science, London: (In press)

Wager, K., Cox, S., 2009. Auricular acupuncture and addiction. Elsevier Science, London.

The Christie NHS Foundation Trust
Wilmslow Rd
Withington
Manchester
M20 4BX
0161 446 8236 or email peter.mackereth@
  Christie.nhs.uk

NHS Stop Smoking Helpline
0800 169 0 169 www.gosmokefree.co.uk
  www.givingupsmoking.co.uk

Pregnancy smoking helpline
0800 169 9169 (12–9 p.m. everyday)

NHS Asian Tobacco Helpline (1–9 p.m.)
  Tuesdays)
Urdu 08001690881 (other language lines
  available)

SMART UK Head Office
27 Park Street
Leamington Spa
Warwickshire
CV32 4QN UK info@smart-uk.com Tel 01926
  311912

Alcoholics Anonymous (AA)
PO BOX 1
Stonebow House York
YO1 2NJ
www.alcohols-anonymous.org.uk

Drinkline – The National Alcohol
  Helpline
0800 917 8282

Al Anon Family Groups UK and Eire
61 Great Dover Street
London
SE1 4YF
Tel: 0207403 0888 www.al-anonuk.org.uk

Narcotics Anonymous (NA) UK Service
  Office
202 City Road
London
EC1V 2PH
020 7251 4007

Talk to Frank
0800 77 66 00; www.talktofrank.co.uk

Reflexology and withdrawal from addictive substances

Reflexology incorporating new techniques

Jill Norfolk • Jan Williamson • Denise Tiran

ABSTRACT

This chapter explores the concept of new developments within reflexology practice, in which experienced practitioners have incorporated new techniques based on the theoretical principles of other complementary therapies. In this chapter we offer three examples: foot-applied Bowen technique (Jill Norfolk), Precision reflexology (Jan Williamson) and Structural reflex zone therapy (Denise Tiran). There are other developments which are not included in this book, but readers are also referred to Chapter 11, in which Gunnell Berry discusses Adapted Reflextherapy, an adaptation which is based on physiotherapy and musculoskeletal function.

KEY WORDS

Synergy, communication, combinations, Bowen technique, Chakra, Precision reflexology, linking, Structural reflex zone therapy.

DOI: 10.1016/B978-0-7020-3167-0.00014-7

INTRODUCTION

Experienced complementary practitioners are constantly developing and refining their practice and expanding their skills in order to increase their repertoire of tools for treatment. An established practitioner comes to appreciate that no single approach, or even one single modality, can be effective for everyone. Some clients respond better to one form of treatment than another, and the needs of each individual can change from session to session. The client–practitioner relationship is significant in determining how well the client will respond to treatment, but the reflexologist may then consider it appropriate to combine the primary method of treatment with different reflexology approaches, or even to incorporate a second therapy, according to the client's overall condition and personal preferences. Each practitioner will use professional knowledge and experience in order to decide which approach to treatment is appropriate for the client. Any changes to existing treatment regimens depend on the establishment of a relationship of mutual trust and respect so that both the client and the therapist feel confident with any adaptations to the treatment intervention. The reflexologist should always involve the client in the process by giving reasons for adopting a new approach, obtaining his or her informed consent to try something new and facilitating the client to evaluate the treatment afterwards.

A combined approach provides additional tools for clinical effectiveness and extra choices for clients. It enables treatment to be client-focused, rather than therapy-focused, a concept which has been discussed in respect of treating pregnant women (Tiran 2009a, b, see also Ch. 9). In clinical practice, particularly that based in NHS institutions or GP practices, clients present with the symptoms inherent in their medical conditions. Unless they have chosen to pay for private reflexology treatment (or other complementary therapy), they have not usually selected that particular therapy, in the same way as a patient does not normally present to the doctor specifically for surgery or medication. What clients/patients require is a resolution to their aches and pains and, although complementary medicine is far more focused on the client–practitioner partnership, which allows clients some autonomy and choice, clients put their trust in the practitioner to decide what is most appropriate for their needs. If this requires a combination of different treatments and the options are explained in full to them, clients will react favourably to receiving therapies which aim to resolve their discomforts.

Utilising several therapies together, or combining aspects of one therapy into the primary choice of treatment modality, also enables a synergistic effect in which the outcome of treatment may be more productive than using a single modality. However, it is essential that practitioners who intend to develop the skills in combining therapies, or introducing new techniques into their general reflexology practice, have consolidated their initial learning and have undertaken appropriate professional education to do so (see Ch. 3). Reflexologists must be experienced enough to understand the effects of their generic reflexology treatment on clients before incorporating new techniques which may cause unanticipated or different effects which could potentially go unrecognised in inexperienced hands. They must also have sound theoretical background knowledge of both the principal style of reflexology and the new techniques they wish to use. In addition, there is a need for evidence to be collated on these new techniques, and on the integrated – or combined – approach to treatment and care.

FOOT-APPLIED BOWEN TREATMENT

The Bowen technique is an individual modality, created from interpretations of the work of Australian Thomas Ambrose Bowen (1916–1982). The basic Bowen move is completely unique and is key to the success of the treatment. Bowen moves are performed over the tendons, connective tissue and the edges of muscles. Bowen technique is non-diagnostic: the client's body is considered to be the ultimate diagnostic machine, perpetually striving to restore and maintain a harmony within itself from the cellular to the whole. Each part of the body already knows its precise function and its relationship to all other parts of the body within the holistic harmonious structure. Bowen technique is a gentle 'baton', which the practitioner uses like a conductor to harmonise and tune the complicated orchestra of the body to allow it to play the symphony of life for which it was created. Bowen practitioners develop an acute sensitivity to soft tissue tension which assists them in making the precise moves with the grace, rhythm, accuracy and gentleness that is the very essence of the Bowen technique.

The concept of combining the principles of reflexology and the procedures of the Bowen technique has not yet been generally accepted, since Bowen technique practitioners consider it to be a stand-alone modality which should never be combined with other work. However, the suggestion to perform Bowen sessions via the reflex points on the feet was triggered by the case of a client who had successfully been receiving regular Bowen sessions for her asthmatic condition, but who then had a car accident which left her with broken ribs. As a result, she was unable to position herself face down on the massage table, and even sitting upright for any length of time was uncomfortable. She was therefore offered the opportunity to recline in a comfortable chair and to receive reflexology treatment instead. However, the client trusted and felt most comfortable with the Bowen work, so the practitioner (the author) made an intuitive and conscious decision that, instead of reflexology treatment, she would apply Bowen moves to the respiratory tract reflex points on the feet. The response was instantaneous: the patient felt a degree of relief from her painful ribs and breathed more easily.

This first experience used a combination of reflexology treatment and Bowen technique, but its success motivated the author to chart the moves of the Bowen procedures on the foot reflex zones, and more recently on the hand reflex zones. The complete Bowen procedure transferred very neatly onto the foot reflex zones, with tiny Bowen moves able to be applied to tendons, muscles and connective tissues of the feet, and treatment achieving a full body-balancing effect. This was then documented so that the findings could be disseminated to other practitioners and taught as a treatment modality in its own right, or as an adjunct to full-body Bowen technique sessions.

It was seen that clients appeared to respond better to this combination treatment than to either of the therapies applied in isolation. Clients with conditions which would normally respond positively to reflexology seemed to respond more rapidly and more positively when Bowen procedures on the feet were applied in place of regular reflexology techniques. Successful outcomes have been achieved for several conditions including frozen shoulder, blocked sinuses which caused headaches, asthma, temporomandibular joint problems, various digestive tract problems, severe heartburn, constipation and irritable bowel syndrome.

POTENTIAL FACTORS BEHIND THE SUCCESS OF FOOT-APPLIED BOWEN TECHNIQUE

There are several factors which may contribute to the success of this modality, possibly making it superior to traditional Bowen techniques for certain conditions. In common with reflexology, sitting face to face with the client means that even the slightest reactions to the Bowen procedures can be detected immediately, and emotional issues frequently surface. This is particularly noticeable with clients who have been treated with Bowen therapy over a prolonged period of time. For some clients it is easier to position themselves in the chair than to attempt to get onto a massage table, for example clients with musculoskeletal disorders, or women who are pregnant. The treatment effects seem to work at a deeper level than Bowen technique alone, accessing all around the muscles, even those not normally accessible on the body's surface, particularly spinal muscles such as the erector spinae, which can visibly relax after the treatment. The glands and endocrine tissues are more accessible via the foot reflex zones, and proportionally they have much more prominence on the feet than via the gross anatomy, and hence hormonal imbalances and digestion issues seem to respond very quickly. Also, many systemic conditions, for example allergic reactions such as headaches, blocked sinuses, etc., are relieved rapidly. Clients who have previously received conventional reflexology have reported that foot-applied Bowen technique feels completely different – more powerful and focused. Many people can correctly identify which part of the body is being working on through its reflex area. Every client, without exception, has reported a deep feeling of relaxation at the end of the session, some even fall into a deep sleep during it.

PRECAUTIONS TO FOOT-APPLIED BOWEN TREATMENT

All the existing contraindications and precautions that apply to reflexology are applicable to the foot-applied Bowen (FAB) method, such as for patients with diabetes, although treatment of the endocrine glands, the lymphatic system and the kidney reflex zones using FAB have proved highly beneficial. When working on a particularly sensitive client, it may be appropriate to leave 2-minute gaps between some of the sequences of moves, as with regular Bowen technique, to determine the extent of the treatment and the level of the client's tolerance to treatment. In particular, the duration of treatment for pregnant women should be reduced as a matter of course, in keeping with reflex zone therapy during pregnancy (see Ch. 9). However, the 2-minute gaps between procedures are not universally needed, perhaps because Bowen work is received by the body remotely, via the reflex zones, and the body is capable of responding appropriately in the same way as with both Bowen therapy and reflexology. In this way, some FAB method applied to the feet or hands at the end of a Bowen session on the body can give some extra emphasis to certain regions and serves as a further trigger to the body's own self-healing capacities.

CASE STUDY 14.1

Beryl was an elderly lady who had been in the care of the social services since the age of 6 due to a rare chromosome disorder called cri du chat syndrome (CDCS), a relatively rare chromosome disorder (chromosome number 5) affecting approximately 1 in 37 000–50 000 live births. At birth, the main clinical diagnostic feature of the syndrome is a high-pitched, monochromatic 'cat-like' cry that is always present in the newborn, but may disappear with age. Other features include a round, full face ('moon face'), widely spread eyes, an extra fold of skin at the inner corners of the eyes (epicanthal folds), a flattened and widened nasal bridge and ears that are positioned low on the head. Most children with CDCS will have feeding problems from birth including failure to thrive, poor sucking and slow weight gain.

When the reflexologist met her, Beryl was in her 70s: her longevity was highly unusual as the average life expectancy of someone with this condition is much shorter, most professional literature on the syndrome referring only to children or babies. It was arranged that she receive reflexology twice a week over a period of several months. On meeting the reflexologist, Beryl had minimal, hard-to-comprehend verbal communication, but complete understanding of everything said and done to her. She could be quite captivating to be around and obviously loved attention paid to her; she was able to communicate pleasure and displeasure, and to indicate any painful sites. Physically, Beryl was confined to a day-bed or a recliner chair with her feet elevated, and could not walk or dress herself. Both arms were permanently bent at the elbow at approximately 40 degrees, and her left leg turned permanently inwards, with the toes hitting the right foot. She complained initially of pain in her right knee, but it was impossible to determine more than just a site of discomfort. Beryl bruised very easily, and the tissues took an extended time to recover.

Foot-applied Bowen therapy was selected as the modality of choice, as it was considered that Bowen procedures would be beneficial, physically and emotionally, but the only easy access to her body was via her feet, legs, arms and hands. Beryl made a real effort to communicate throughout the sessions, which apparently indicated a positive acceptance on her part of the work being done to her; if unhappy, she would have just remained totally silent. During the first eight sessions a giant television with the volume turned up loudly was located in the room, and care home staff instructed that it should remain on for the benefit of other residents. These were hardly ideal conditions in which to treat Beryl. Later, the television needed repairing and a radio was found instead, which provided Beryl with the opportunity to sing along during her foot treatment and her ankles and legs would move in time to the music. Using foot-applied Bowen treatment, Beryl received Bowen relaxation procedures and specific Bowen techniques on the foot reflex zones for the sacrococcygeal and kidney areas, the respiratory tract, the temporomandibular joint, knees, hamstring muscles and shoulders and elbows. Not all reflex zones were treated at every session.

There was a general overall improvement in Beryl's condition which was recognised by the nursing staff in the unit. She became more flexible, her arms became almost straightened, her hips straightened fully, allowing both legs to rest side by side, she stopped reporting pain in her knee and she seemed to become much less prone to bruising. She also became more communicative, appeared happier and became increasingly animated even trying to play 'air guitar' to some rock-and-roll songs, which made her laugh out loud. Beryl passed away very peacefully in her sleep a few months later but the nursing staff and social services staff both reported that the reflexology/foot-applied Bowen treatments had helped her immensely in the last few months of her life.

PRECISION REFLEXOLOGY

Precision Reflexology has the same rationale as other forms of reflexology in that it focuses on stimulating reflex points on the feet in the belief that these have a connection with related parts of the body. The healing process is considered to result from restoration and maintenance of good health within the entire system.

THE LINKING TECHNIQUE

However, in addition to conventional reflexology treatment, Precision Reflexology incorporates a unique technique called 'linking', enabling the practitioner to connect to the subtle energy of each client. Over the years, many therapists who have qualified in generic reflexology have incorporated the 'linking' technique of precision work into their own practice. A specific Precision Reflexology chart has been devised but is used purely as a guide, because the philosophy of Precision Reflexology is that students are taught to recognise the reflex points by their sense of touch. Skilled practitioners can identify and differentiate between the relevant reflexes by the responses that they feel in their fingers. This is especially true for the 'links', each one of which has its own character so that the therapist can locate it through his or her fingers rather than using a foot chart. In this way, it could be argued that, whichever chart a reflexologist uses, Precision techniques can be incorporated into the reflexology treatment. The simplicity of Precision linking means that it can easily be incorporated into any reflexology procedures without practitioners needing to make dramatic changes to their existing routine. Some people choose to complete their treatment and then add any appropriate links at the end of the session. Others find it easier to include the links within the treatment, applying each one as they work the relevant area.

Precision Reflexology requires practitioners to have an awareness of the body's subtle energy but this does not mean that it should present challenges for their own belief systems. Linking uses a light touch to connect two, three or four defined reflex points in order to add power and precision to the overall treatment. It is believed that a firm touch prevents the energetic response from being felt, and experience appears to indicate that strong physical pressure negates the holistic nature of the modality. Precision methods are especially suitable for clients who are vulnerable and weak, either physically or emotionally, and those who prefer a gentle touch. Experienced practitioners will use their professional judgement to determine who they think will respond favourably to a light touch. This approach is not invasive and is 'client-friendly', with progress through the course of treatment proceeding at a pace suitable for the individual. This gentle approach also reflects the nature of the consultation process, in which clients are given an element of choice and the practitioner merely facilitates the opportunity for the body to heal itself, using its own innate intelligence.

THE EAST–WEST LINK

Whilst Precision Reflexology is Western in application, it is also true to the Eastern origins of reflexology, which recognises that illness is an imbalance of energy and that treatment aims to help restore balance to the entire system in order to improve homeostasis. The unique nature of Precision work is that it offers the opportunity to connect *directly* to the energetic system of the body, to adjust it and to harmonise it within itself and with the world surrounding each recipient. Each practitioner will obviously have her or his own way of expressing this energy; they may use terms such as prana (as in the Yogic system), or Chi (as in Chinese medicine) or Vital Force (as in homeopathy). Whatever terminology is used, it refers to the system which operates within each of us in a multidirectional network of communication that works on physical, emotional, mental and spiritual levels.

Precision Reflexology may also involve the use of chakras, centres of energy believed to be within the body and which can offer an explanation of the concept of subtle energy (Ozaniec 1990). The relevance to the linking method is that each chakra is thought to have a physical counterpart within the endocrine system. Since there are also Precision links associated with each endocrine gland, linking allows direct access to the subtle energy of the body. Each chakra is thought to represent different aspects of the individual's unique personality (Table 14.1). Chakra work can provide a very practical way to work holistically and offers a means of working with a concept that is often seen as being esoteric and difficult to define. This aspect of Precision work will not be acceptable for all practitioners, but for some it offers an added dimension to treatments.

Table 14.1 *Relationships between precision reflexology and chakras*

Chakra	Physical aspect	Non-physical aspect
Crown	Pineal gland	Spiritual awareness
Brow	Pituitary gland	Intuition
Throat	Thyroid gland	Communication
Heart	Thymus gland	Relationships
Solar plexus	Pancreas	Confidence
Sacral	Adrenal glands	Courage
Root	Gonads	Vitality

Reflexology incorporating new techniques

Recent developments in Precision Reflexology further incorporate this connection with the chakra system and have led to a system of Advanced Precision Reflexology which encompasses a variety of modalities that resonate with each chakra in turn. This also involves the client in using a range of self-help procedures. Practitioners wishing to progress to the Advanced techniques should have a basic understanding of energy work, basic Precision Reflexology and the linking techniques.

EXAMPLES OF LINKING

'Linking' involves simultaneously holding two or more previously identified reflex points on the feet to add strength and definition to the reflexology treatment. As the link is held, the practitioner pauses and is aware of responses that can be felt on each of the points. The responses vary enormously from one individual to another but may feel like a small tingle, a vibrant pulse, a hot or cold sensation or an intense feeling of well-being and relaxation beneath the practitioner's fingers. Often, there is a distinction between the points, with one feeling more energetic than the other, which should equalise as the link is held. The duration for which each link is held is determined individually and it can take several sessions to achieve a sense of equilibrium. Initially, it is sufficient just to be aware of any change in the vibrations that are felt. Existing clients need to be made aware of the stillness that is involved in the holding of this technique and that changes in well-being may be achieved after one session, or that it may take a course of treatment. The therapeutic responses can either be an improvement in physical symptoms or a positive change in emotional or spiritual issues. The effects produced range from energising and uplifting to calming and relaxing and can vary from one client to another or between treatments in one client. There are defined sets of links, each with the potential to produce particular effects and with their own specific applications. Each link has its own characteristics. Some of them can provoke feelings of being expansive and free, others of deep relaxation and some can initiate a powerful emotional response, but it is not suitable to use all the links within a single consultation, nor for all clients. Practitioners use their expertise in order to determine which links to use. Experienced practitioners can use this approach with accuracy and sensitivity (Williamson 1999).

EXAMPLES OF LINKS

There is a full range of links which connect to the skeletal, endocrine, respiratory, digestive, circulatory, nervous, immune, muscular and reproductive systems of the body. It is not appropriate to describe each of them in this chapter, but two are detailed here in order to illustrate the method.

Neck-to-jaw link

The reflex point for the fifth cervical vertebra is linked to the jaw reflex point (on the inside of the big toe) (Fig.14.1A). It has been found to be most

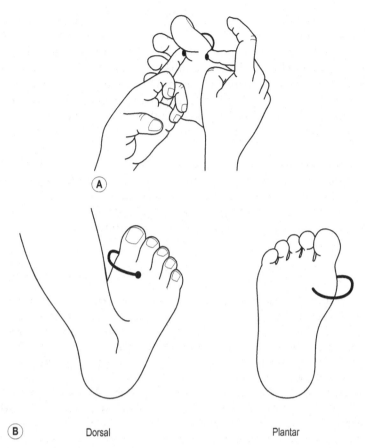

| B | Dorsal | Plantar |

FIG. 14.1 A,B Diagrams to show linking in precision reflexology.

effective if the practitioner uses the thumb or middle finger, and both hands. This neck-to-jaw link can be effective for any neck condition, pain and tension in the jaw or tension headaches. The practitioner may feel a pulsating sensation in either or both of the points. Often, heat is felt by either the therapist or the client. The client may report feeling a connection running through, or around, the big toe and sometimes a warmth or pulsation in the neck. People who have neck problems often find the reflex point for the neck is extremely tender to touch and this link provides an effective method of treatment whilst using a light touch. In addition, this link is also responsive for people who are very 'driven' personalities, who like being in control and who find it difficult to relax. Over time, such people can begin to respond positively to this intervention.

Thyroid link

This is located by holding the central point of the thyroid reflex on the plantar aspect of the foot with the thumb of one hand and a point immediately above, on the dorsal aspect, with the middle finger of the other hand

(Fig. 14.1B). The dorsal point is held still while the practitioner works the whole of the plantar thyroid reflex. Often the practitioner feels a strong pulsation or tingling sensation and the client may report a tender, pulsing, rod-like feeling between the two points. This link can be equally effective for an underactive or an overactive thyroid gland because it aims to restore balance. It can also be helpful for clients with low energy levels and with metabolic imbalances. It assists the natural function of the thyroid gland as it helps to adjust the calcium levels in the body, together with the parathyroid glands.

The chakra counterpart for the thyroid gland is the throat chakra, which has, as its main characteristic, communication. The author has observed many cases in which this link has been effective in helping clients who have communication problems; often a response occurs naturally over the course of treatment without the need for discussion (see Case Study 14.2).

CASE STUDY 14.2

A 45-year-old woman, who was married, with two teenage children, and who worked fulltime as a teacher, presented with tension headaches and insomnia. On examination of the feet, the neck reflexes were extremely tender and tense and the neck-to-jaw link was applied to both feet. The thyroid link was also found to be very erratic, although there were no apparent physical symptoms to account for this, but each time the thyroid link was held the client reported feeling very relaxed. A course of six full Precision Reflexology treatments was given over a period of 3 months, when the client reported a marked reduction in both the frequency and severity of the headaches. Her sleeping patterns had also improved. In addition, she also explained to the reflexologist that her working situation had improved because she had been able to talk to her head of department about some issues that had been bothering her. She had not previously mentioned this communication problem but she now felt that her stress levels were markedly reduced because she had been able to take the initiative to resolve her problem.

STRUCTURAL REFLEX ZONE THERAPY

PHYSIOLOGICAL BASIS OF STRUCTURAL REFLEX ZONE THERAPY

Structural reflex zone therapy (SRZT) is an adaptation from reflex zone therapy devised by Tiran (2004). It builds on a variation of reflexology, that of reflex zone therapy originally developed by Hanne Marquardt (1983) and refined by Lett (2000). However, SRZT also applies the principles of osteopathy, using the reflex zones on the feet as a medium through which musculoskeletal (M-S) misalignments can be rectified or discomforts arising from M-S misalignment can be treated. Osteopathy (and chiropractic) is based on the principle that the

M-S system is the main supportive framework of the body, with the body's soft tissues attached either internally or externally to the framework, and that changes in anatomical structure will lead to physiological dysfunction and altered homeostasis, potentially triggering chemical, neurological, electrical or biomechanical problems. SRZT, like osteopathy, focuses on the inter-relationship between the structure and function of the body. The reflex zones on the feet, particularly those for the M-S system, are thus manipulated to correct or reduce anatomical imbalances which may have contributed to physiological disorders or disease.

Although SRZT has not so far been formally researched, it is based on the solid scientific foundations of anatomy, physiology and neurological links, and practice of this type of therapy thus requires a comprehensive knowl-edge of the M-S system, as well as refined clinical skills relating to reflex zone therapy. An appreciation of the differences between generic reflexology and reflex zone therapy is essential, including the different techniques which are used in treatment, variations in the charts and theories and awareness of the reactions which may occur during, after and between treatments. Careful history-taking is fundamental to any clinical practice and in SRZT includes a systematic analysis of the client's history and current condition in relation to the M-S system.

TREATMENT TECHNIQUES

Treatment with reflex zone therapy in general, and SRZT in particular, is not performed for relaxation (although this may occur as a result of the treat-ment). The treatment session may be of short duration, sometimes lasting as little as 10 minutes, and usually incorporates a range of techniques aimed at treating the symptoms and the cause of the presenting condition. This may include stimulation (a precise clinical technique which differs from the 'stim-ulation' performed in a general relaxation reflexology treatment: see Ch. 7), sedation, holding and other techniques as appropriate. In addition, SRZT incorporates specialised manipulative techniques designed to realign the reflex zones corresponding to the M-S system, in the same way as an osteo-path would use manipulative techniques on the whole body. This leads to a much more dynamic treatment than is used in many forms of reflexology, and is diametrically opposed to gentle forms such as Precision, Morrell or Gentle Touch™ reflexology.

To date, SRZT has been used in the author's own clinical field, namely maternity care, but could be applied to other clinical specialities. It does, how-ever, require the practitioner to have a deep understanding of the relevant anatomy, physiology and pathology related to the client's condition, as well as how the therapy may interact with any conventional medical treatment. For a comprehensive exploration of SRZT applied to pregnancy and child-birth, see Tiran 2009a,b. The effectiveness of SRZT has anecdotally been dem-onstrated in over 5000 women treated by the author, sometimes resolving intransigent problems such as backache or 'morning sickness' in pregnancy (see Case Study 14.3 and Ch. 9).

Reflexology incorporating new techniques

CASE STUDY 14.3

'Morning sickness' is caused primarily by the pregnancy hormones, oestrogen and chorionic gonadotrophin, although other factors such as tiredness, hunger, stress and illness will exacerbate it. However, research by the author over a 15-year period suggests that there is a higher incidence of severe 'morning sickness' in women with a history of neck, back or jaw problems, particularly conditions such as whiplash injury from a road accident or following traumatic dental surgery. Existing symptoms of nausea and vomiting in pregnancy will be compounded by the impact of the expanding uterus on the upper gastrointestinal tract and compromised biomechanical movement in the diaphragm, thorax and upper abdomen, whilst tension in the cervical spine may aggravate the vagus nerve, further exacerbating nausea.

Georgina was expecting her second baby, having had a normal pregnancy and birth with her son, three years ago. Since his birth she had suffered a displaced intervertebral disc (slipped disc) at the level of the third lumbar vertebra, which happened as she bent down to lift a casserole out of the oven. This had led to ongoing backache, sciatica and headaches. Although she had not experienced more than occasional nausea in her first pregnancy, she felt extremely unwell this time, and was referred to the midwife-reflexologist when she was 17 weeks pregnant. On examination, her feet were swollen around the reflex zone for the spine, especially the upper thoracic and lumbosacral areas, and the hip zones were tender to touch, notably on the right. The reflex zones for the oesophagus and cardiac sphincter of the stomach were also very sensitive, suggesting heartburn, which Georgina confirmed.

SRZT was performed by focusing on the reflex zones for the spine, sedating the third to fifth lumbar vertebrae, the sacrum and also the twelfth thoracic vertebra, from which a neurological link to the vomiting centre in the brain often exacerbates nausea. Sedation to the hip reflex zone, particularly the sacroiliac joint zone, was also applied. Further, sedation of the symptomatic portion of the reflex zone for the oesophagus was given, as well as sedation of the cardiac sphincter zone, until Georgina could no longer feel any tenderness in these areas. Manipulation, using a dynamic twisting movement to the entire length of the spine zones was then performed until a 'cracking' sound was elicited, indicating a release of tension. At this point, Georgina reported that she felt less nauseous, and that a headache she had had on arrival had resolved. The 'hands-on' part of the treatment lasted 6 minutes. Georgina was given a follow-up appointment for the following week, but cancelled 2 days before, stating that she was much improved and had managed to attend her son's nursery school play.

CONCLUSION

Reflexology is a constantly evolving profession, within which there are now many different styles, specialisms and theories. The practice of experienced therapists often reveals new ways of working, especially when those practitioners have specialised in a particular field or when they have a broad knowledge of both conventional healthcare and of other complementary therapies. Intuitive practitioners are alert to nuances in the feet, including internal energies and links between one part of the body and another, and can build on their findings and experience to develop additional elements of the therapy. This chapter has discussed just three new forms of reflexology, in which aspects of other therapies are incorporated, either at a theoretical level, or through the precise techniques used. These now need to be formally evaluated and documented in order to assess whether or not the results ensuing from use of these therapies are transferable.

REFERENCES

Lett, A., 2000. Reflex zone therapy for health professionals. Churchill Livingstone, Edinburgh.

Marquardt, H., 1983. Reflex zone therapy of the feet. Thorson Wellingborough Mitchell & Cormack, Edinburgh.

Norfolk, J., 2005. FAB method – a training and instruction manual. Jill Norfolk Complementary Therapies. http://www.fabmethod.co.uk http://www.criduchat.co.uk/diagnosis.html.

Ozaniec, N., 1990. The chakras. Element Books, Dorset.

Tiran, D., 2004. Nausea and vomiting in pregnancy: an integrated approach to care. Elsevier Science, Edinburgh.

Tiran, D., 2009a. Reflexology for pregnancy and childbirth: a definitive guide for healthcare professionals. Elsevier, Edinburgh.

Tiran, D., 2009b. Structural reflex zone therapy in pregnancy and childbirth: a new approach. Complement. Ther. Clin. Pract. 15 (4), 234–238.

Williamson, J., 1999. A guide to precision reflexology. Quay Books, Wiltshire.

FURTHER READING

Mitchell, A., Cormack, M., 1998. The therapeutic relationship in complementary health care. Churchill Livingstone, Edinburgh.

USEFUL RESOURCES

www.expectancy.co.uk.
www.precisionreflexology.com.

www.fabmethod.co.uk

INDEX

Note: Page numbers followed by *b* indicate boxes; *f* figures; *t* tables.

INDEX

Printed in the United States
By Bookmasters